Pathology atlas of nasopharyngeal carcinoma(NPC) and other diseases of nose and nasopharynx

鼻、鼻咽疾病病理图谱

Editor in chief: Lu Xian-yu
Translator: Hou Jing-hui

天津科技翻译出版公司出版

图书在版编目(CIP)数据

鼻、鼻咽疾病病理图谱:英文/陆献瑜编著. --
天津:天津科技翻译出版公司,2010.4
ISBN 978-7-5433-2691-0

Ⅰ.①鼻… Ⅱ.①陆… Ⅲ.①鼻咽肿瘤—病理学—图谱—英文 Ⅳ.①R739.63-64

中国版本图书馆 CIP 数据核字(2010)第 055303 号

出　　版:天津科技翻译出版公司
出 版 人:蔡 颢
地　　址:天津市南开区白堤路 244 号
邮政编码:300192
电　　话:022-87894896
传　　真:022-87895650
网　　址:www.tsttpc.com
印　　刷:山东临沂新华印刷集团有限公司
发　　行:全国新华书店
版本记录:880×1230　32 开本　4.25 印张　180 千字
2010 年 4 月第 1 版　2010 年 4 月第 1 次印刷
定价:45.00 元

Introduction of editor-in-chief

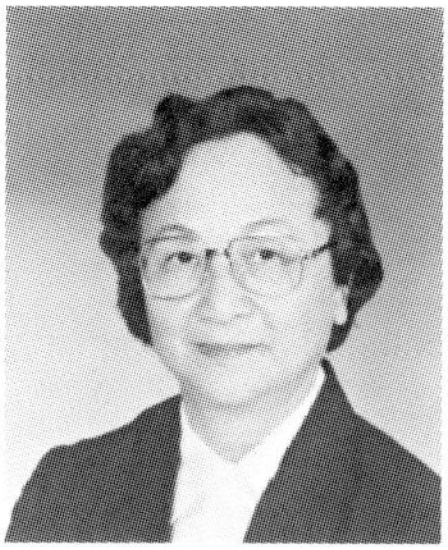

Lu Xian-yu, Professor of Pathology at Sun Yat-sen University Cancer Center, was born in December 1928. She has been engaged in clinical diagnosis; teaching and research work for several decades, and made a great achievement.

Prof. Lu worked precisely and accumulated abundant experience on diagnosis of difficult cases. She differentiated many specious cancer cases and rectified many wrong diagnoses to avoid unnecessary radiotherapy, chemo-therapy and radical operations. Also she compiled textbooks and held many training lessons of tumors. A lot of professionals specializing in pathology have been trained. Prof. Lu devoted herself to the research of nasopharynx, liver, breast, thyroid carcinomas and malignant lymphoma. Remarkable successes have been achieved. 58 research papers were published. She compiled the electrical teaching material of clinical pathology which was entitled "Nasopharyngeal Carcinomas, Nasal and other Nasopharyngeal Diseases" and won the 2nd prize of audio-visual aid textbook of higher education. She also took part in the compiling of "The Clinical and Experimental

Research of Nasopharyngeal Carcinoma", which got the 1st prize of the National Science and Technology Publication. The finding of four pigs with early NPC out of 17923 pigs made she got the 3rd Science and Research award of Guangzhou. The research papers about nasopharynx, liver, breast thyroid carcinomas and malignant lymphoma also won 2nd, 3rd, and 4th Research Prize of Guangdong province, Guangzhou respectively.

Prof. Lu enjoys a special allowance granted by the State Council of Chinese Government.

Hou Jing-hui

Preface

Sun Yat-sen University Cancer Center is a well known institution for diagnosis, treatment and research work on nasopharyngeal carcinomas (NPC). The affiliated hospital has admitted and treated thousands of patients coming from all over the country and the southeastern Asia. In order to providing more facilities and references in contributing to training of medical professionals and to raise further the diagnosis and research level of NPC, the authors compiled this atlas by collecting photographs with either gross or microscopic findings from 211 248 biopsies and 8,848 autopsies. Among them, a few cases are from Sun Yat-sen College of Medical Sciences. We hope it will enrich further the documents of pathology, oncology and otorhino laryngology.

Prof. Liang Bo-qiang is one of the founders of pathology in China. He had initiated the work on study/diagnosis/treatment of NPC in China. He had made great pioneer achievements in the field of histopathological classification, biological behavior, origin of NPC and put forward the Liang's classification of NPC, which is significant for further investigation of NPC. Hundred thousands of biopsies and autopsies had been reported according to Liang's classification for several decades, which has become a routine classification for NPC clinically. The NPC cases reported in this atlas were classified under the principle of Liang's classification.

This atlas serves as a reference book for teaching, clinical practice and research programs of NPC in pathology or otorhinolaryngology of medical colleges, hospitals and institutions. It is hard to avoid oversight, criticism and correction are welcome.

Thanks for the help of Prof. She Ming-peng, Zhen Yong-su, Zhong Shi-zhen, Zeng Yi-xin, Wu Qiu-liang. Also thanks to Prof. Sun Zhen-quan and Zhu Jia-zhen for providing some their precious pictures.

Lu Xian–yu ***Editor–in–chief***

2008

Contents

Section 1 General outline

Contents

Section 2 Pathology atlas

1 General outline

1. The pathologic category of Nasopharyngeal carcinoma (NPC)

Any malignant tumor which originates from the epithelium of nasopharynx including the tubular glands and acinus under the mucosa are termed as nasopharyngeal carcinoma (NPC). Histologically, the mucosa locating near by the oral pharynx, the lower half of the posterior wall, the lateral and inferior walls of nasopharynx is covered by squamous epithelium while the area near by the posterior nares is covered by pseudostratified ciliated columnar cell epithelium. Flat shaped transitional cells and squamous cell islands are obtained at the border between the squamous and columnar cell epithelia. There are cuboidal epithelial cells of excreting snot (nasal discharge) and columnar epithelial cells lining the gland tubules underneath the nasopha-ryngeal mucoas. All these epithelial cells might be infected or undergoing malignant change by repeated stimulation of certain pathogens or carcinogenic factors. Carcinomas originating from different epithelial cells might give a different pathological feature and so to have a different corresponding therapeutic regimen. For example, the morphology of well-differentiated carcinoma cells is somewhat close to normal epithelial cells, such as keratinizing squamous cell carcinoma, basal cell carcinoma, papillary adenocarcinoma originating from the columnar cell of gland tubules, and adenoid cystic carcinoma originating from the gland acinar cells. All of these cells are insensitive to radiation therapy, so that, it's important to have an earlier pathologic diagnosis and an effective corresponding therapeutic plan.

Tumors originating from other tissue in nasopharynx are not termed as NPC. The malignant tumors originating from lymph tissue under the nasopharyngeal mucosa are called lymphoma, of which the principle treatment is chemotherapy. The malignant tumors originating from soft tissue or blood vessels under the nasopharyngeal mucosa are called sarcoma and the therapeutic principles are different. Therefore, in addition to different types of NPC, the author had also enumerated the benign and malignant tumors of both nasopharynx and nose as well as different kinds of inflammatory and tumor-like lesions for differential diagnosis. It's important to ensure the biopsy diagnosis before to make a therapeutic regimen for the cancer patients.

2. Problems concerning pathohistological classification of NPC

The principle of histopathological classification for NPC of this atlas is according to Liang Bo-qiang's histopathological classification. In order to make an easlier comprehension of this classification for the readers, the authors have listed the latest version of WHO's histopathological classification[3] in contrast as follows:

Histopathological classification of NPC

(based on Liang Bo-qiang's histopathological classification)

2.1 Undifferentiated Carcinoma (Fig.61–64)

Pleomorphic cell carcinoma (large cell type and small cell type)

2.2 Poorly differentiated Carcinoma

2.2.1 Giant round cell carcinoma (distant metastasis common) (Fig.68–71)

2.2.2 Spindle cell carcinoma (with a tendency of invading base of the skull commonly) (Fig.65–67)

2.2.3 Squamous cell carcinoma grade III (invasion of base of skull and distant metastasis) (Fig.54– 60)

2.2.4 Clear cell carcinoma(Fig.79–82)

2.2.5 Mixed–cell Poorly differentiated Carcinoma (Fig.87)

2.3. Well differentiated Carcinoma.

2.3.1 Squamous cell carcinoma grade I (Fig.48–51)

2.3.2 Squamous cell carcinoma grade II (Fig.52)

2.3.3 Adenosquamous carcinoma(Fig.85)

2.3.4 Columnar cell adenocarcinoma (including tubular adenocarcinoma and Papillary adenocarcinoma) (图 88, 89, 99–103)

2.3.5 Cuboidal cell carcinoma (including Acinar cell carcinoma) (Fig.91–98)

2.3.6 Mucoepidermoid carcinoma(Fig.104,105)

2.3.7 Adenoid cystic carcinoma(Fig.106–117)

2.3.8 Basal cell carcinoma(Fig.46,47)

Since the photographs published in this atlas are the representative cases of NPC which were selected from 211,248 biopsy and 8,848 autopsy cases, so that the number of types classified was expanded and more than that in the before. Some tumors are rarely seen in the past, such as adenosquamous carcinoma, cuboidal acinar cell carcinoma that originate from the gland acinus and tubules under the nasopharyngeal mucosa, as well as adenoid cystic carcinoma. These tumors are not sensitive to radiation therapy and metastasis also rarely occurs. In figures'110–113, the primary adenoid cystic carcinoma was resistant to radiation therapy, and unfortunately in this case, another malignant fibrous histocytoma developed in stroma after radiation therapy. It seems important to emphasize that for those well differentiated and non-metastasized NPC, completely removal of the primary tumor mass is recommended and further therapeutic regimen is suggested in trial.

Basing on the data of analysis of 50 NPC autopsy cases reported by Liang Bo-qiang et al[2], types or features of the secondary or metastatic tumors might be different from that of the original ones. For instance, Squamous cell carcinoma or spindle cell carcinoma originally seen in biopsy specimens might be changing into pleomorphic cell carcinoma in the metastatic nodules and occasionally, different diagnosis might appear in the autopsy findings. Recently immunohistochemical detection confirmed that cytokeratin (CK)is positive in spindle cell carcinoma, pleomorphic cell carcinoma and most giant round cell carcinoma indicating that NPC mostly originate from squamous cell epithelium or from malignant change of squamous cell metaplasia of the columnar epithelium[4-6]。

Basal cells of squamous epithelium as showed in Fig.s.68 and 69 and cells in stratum basalis of the gland tubules lining with columnar cells as showed in Fig.70, all are able undergoing atypical hyperplasia; then malignant change to transform into giant round cell carcinoma. The author considered that giant round cell carcinoma belonged to an undifferentiated type. It might originate from cells of stratum basalis of squamous epithelium or from the basal cells of glands and tubules.

【Remarks 1】the author considered that the term “differentiated non-keratinizing carcinoma” raised in WHO NPC pathological classification, reflected the clinical feature, and seem worth to be preserved. Practically, malignant tumors occur from transitional cells of squamous epithelium and well-differentiated columnar epithelium. They are non-keratinizing, mitosis scanty, and developed slowly, similar to lympho-epithelioma or the transitional cell carcinoma.

【Remarks 2】WHO histological classification of tumours of the nasopharynx is too simple to express cytomorphological characters and is not in favour to clinic study of treatment pro-

WHO NPC pathohistological classification[3] tumours of the nasopharynx	
Malignant epithelia tumours	
NPC	
Non-keratinizing carcinoma	8027/3
Keratinizing squamous cell carcinoma	8071/3
Basaloid squamous cell carcinoma	8083/3
Nasopharyngeal papillary adenocarcinoma	8206/3
Salivary gland-type Carcinoma	

jects of all kinds of NPC. Therefore, cytomorphological characters and differentiated degree of cancer cells are taken as the base of histological classification in this book.

【Remarks 3】In order to express cytomorphological characterstics in favour to cilinical study of treatment projects of all kinds of NPC, cytomorphological characteristics and differentiated degree of cancer cells are taken as the base of histological classification in this book. Moreover, Liang's classification depended on lots of biopsy and anatomy datas is recommended. For example, giant round cell carcinoma of the nasopharynx was used to being called clear nuclear cell carcinoma. The author considers that the nucleus of most adenocarcinoma nuclear is clear; however it has been confirmed that cases of giant round cell carcinoma of the nasopharynx may originate from glandular and squamous epithelia (see Fig. 68–71).

3. Clinical symptoms and diagnosis of NPC

3.1 Symptoms of first visit to a doctor

If mucosa is involved in early stage, nasal hemorrhage and blood sputum may emerge. Nasal obstruction and nasal hemorrhage may appear if parietal wall or nearly posterior naris is involved. Headache, tinnitus, hypoacusis, exudative tympanitis may appear if parietal wall of nasopharynx, auditory tube, protuberance and pharyngeal recess is involved. Some patients didn't have any auris and nasus symptoms. They didn't see a doctor until they had cervical lumps of lymph nodes, or diplopic, goggle-eye, exophthalmus, hypoacusis and one-side temporal, parietal or/and occipital migraine due to the base of skull is invaded.

3.2 Auris and nasus symptoms

Because of NPC invading, enlarging and projecting from surface, patients commonly have purulent and bloody snot due to infection, except nasal hemorrhage for ulcerated, nasal obstruction and tinnitus. Few patients with NPC under mucosa had nasal hemorrhage. If olfactory nerves involved, patients may have hyposmia or anosmia; if Ⅷ pair of cranial nerves involved, patients may have deaf and vertigo.

3.3 Eyes symptoms

NPC may invade the basal skull and cavernous sinus region, and damage the cranial nerves. For example, if trochlear nerve (Ⅳ pair of cranial nerves)is damaged, superior oblique muscle is involved, the patients will have problem of depression in nasal–down direction. If oculomotor nerver (Ⅲ pair of cranial nerves) is damaged, superior rectus muscle, inferior rectus muscle, medial rectus muscle and inferior oblique muscles will be involved, the eyes may be fixed except abduction. If levator palpebrae muscle is involved, patient may have ptosis (blepharoptosis). When the sphincter muscles are involved, pupil dilatation may present. Since abducens nerves (VI pair of cranial nerves) pass a comparatively long distance and through the region that NPC oftens invade, they usually are affected early and result in paralytic diplopia as the first symptom. The patient often go to see oculist first. If NPC invades sphenoid bone, sphenoidal sinus, posterior ethmoidal cells, hypophysial fossa upwards, the region between optic chiasm and optic foramen can be invaded, the patients would have partial blindness and monocular or binocular blindness with optic nerve damage. Optic nerve atrophy may be seen by fundus examination.

NPC could invade orbit through many routes: it can enter the orbit through inferior and superior orbital fissure; come into pterygopalatine fossa along pterygoid canal; enter inner orbit though orbital apex. Posterior ethmoidal cells are involved through posterior naris, thus entering the orbit. If areas around auditory tube are involved frequently, thus invading petrosphenoidal space along fasciae and Ⅲ, Ⅳ and Ⅴ pairs of cranial nerves, the patients may have paralysis of eye movement. What's more, if trigeminal nerve or optic nerve is involved, the patients may have sensory disturbance of nasociliary nerve, eyeball, face, nasal cavity mucosa, lacrimal gland and upper eyelid. Finally, the patients may become blind in one or both eyes. If cervical sympathetic ganglia is involved, the patient may have Horner's Sign, which includes myosis, blepharophimosis and endoophthalmos. If NPC enters the orbit by way of extracranial passageway, the patients may have exophthalmia first, may be with or without cranial nerves symptoms.

3.4 Headache

Headache is one of the more common symptoms of NPC. It may be the earliest or unique symptom. Statistically 68.6% of the 1000 cases in the Tumor Hospital of Sun Yat-sen University complained of headache. Headache that appears in the early stage may be neurovascular reflex headache, or due to the stimulation of the first peripheral branch of trigeminal nerve, or related to backflow obstruction because of tumor internal cervical nerve compressed by. The headache is more common in single temporal, parietal or/and occipital region. The places of hemicrania are relatively steady. In the later stage the patients' neurogenic headache would be much more serious due to the involvement of basicranial bones, also associated with corresponding symptoms of every pair of nerves involved. However, headache would dissapear if tumor involvement paralyed trigeminal nerve, while the symptoms of other pairs of involved nerves still exist.

3.5 The symptoms of mouth and other cranial nerves invided

If Ⅶ pair of cranial nerves (facial nerve) are involved, facial expression muscle may cause disappearence of frontal wrinkle, incompletely closed eyes, nasolabial sulcus shoaling and underlip deflexion. If (one side) IX pair of cranial nerves (glossopharyngeal nerve) are involved, patients may have sensory disturbance of the pharynx and posterio third of the tongue, secretory disturbance of parotid, palatine arches caved in. If X pair of cranial nerves (pneumogastric nerve) are involved, the patients may have anesthesia of hypopharynx and larynx, and that food may be aspirated into the trachea may cause tussis, voice hoarseness, vocal cords paralysis and sensory disturbanc of tragus's skin. If XI pair of cranial nerves(accessorius nerve), are involved, patients' trapezius muscle and sternocleidomastoid muscle may become atrophic and patients may shrug weakly. If XII pair of cranial nerves (hypoglossal nerve), are involved, patients may have unilateral tougue atrophy, and deviation towards the affected side.[6,7]

3.6 The symptyoms of basicranial bones invaded

79% of basicranial bones destroyed have headache, and 21% have no headache. 70% of patients with symptoms of III, IV, V, VI pairs of cranial nerves involved, will have basicranial bones destroyed. Most patients with descending-type NPC invading their cervical lymph nodes do not have basicranial bones destoyed.[6]

3.7 Enlargement of cervical lymph nodes

The metastatic ratio of cervical lymph nodes in NPC is

very high. According to the statistics provided by the Tumor Hospital of Sun Yat-sen University, of the 1000 NPC cases, the metastatic ratio of cervical lymph nodes is 78.9%, and the metastatic ratio of bilateral cervical lymph nodes is 34.1%. Metastatic ratio of NPC in parietal and basal walls is higher. Usually metastasis of parietal and basal walls is the primary symptom which precedes the symptoms of auris and nasus. Of the 1000 cases, the metastatic ratio of NPC in parietal and basal walls is 45.3%, while primay focus was not found in 18 cases (1.8%). It is possible that the primary focus is under mucosa near the pharyngeal recess of the prominance posterosuperior to the auditory tube. So some patients' primary symptom was the enlargement of cervical lymph nodes. Therefore, the nasopharynx of all patients who have enlargement of cervical lymph nodes should be checked. Enlargement of superior deep anterior cervical lymph nodes (under posterior belly of digastric muscle) or posterior cervical lymph nodes (under apex of papillary muscles and deep surface of sternocleidomastoid muscles) may occur first. If the patient's primary focus is located behind nasopharyngeal cavity, enlargement of accessor lymph nodes of posterior triangle of neck may occur firstly[7].

According to lymph drainage of nasopharyngeal cavity, enlargement of retropharyngeal and parapharyngeal lymph nodes may occur firstly; pharyngorhinoscopy shows retropharyngeal mucosa upheaving. If Ⅸ, Ⅹ, Ⅺ, and XII pairs of cranial nerves are involved, enlargement of retropharyngeal lymph nodes should be suspected as the cause. Metastasis of lymph nodes of descending NPC often occurs earlier than that of ascending NPC. According to the statistics of the Tumor Hospital of Sun Yat-sen University, of the 1000 cases, the metastatic ratio of one-side cervical lynph nodes is 43.3%, whereas the metastatic ratio of two-ide cervical lymph nodes was 34.1%. In ascending NPC, squamous cell carcinoma grade I and grade II of NPC usually fewer cases have metastasis, with their ratio being 21.1%.Cervical lymph nodes through thoracic duct communicate with supraclavicular cervical large veins, so cancer cells enter into the blood vessels by this way and distant metastasis may occur. Autopsy showed that the metastatic ratio was 76%[8], and most mestastatic focuses are in bone, lung and liver.

Radiograph shows osteolytic, osteoblastic or mixed focus. Osteoblastic focus appears an even and dense image.Mixed-type appears mottling, radial or pectinal neogenetic bone, mostly seen in thoracic and cervical vertebrae. In the early stage of metastasis in liver, lungs and mediastinum, the patients have no symptoms. In the later stage, the patients may have hemoptysis, chest pain, hepatomegaly and hepatalgia, and mediastinal lymph radiograph may show nodular image, B-ultrasound and CT are helpful for diagnosis.

3.8 Problems of NPC early diagnosis

NPC early diagnosis can improve NPC treatment ratio. In early stage, NPC is limited in nasopharyngeal cavity, basicranial bones, cranial nerves and cervical nodes are all free from NPC no metastasis exist in other distant organs. For many years only 3%~6% of patients with stage I NPC were definitely diagnosed per year in Tumor Hospital of Sun Yat-sen University. The cure treatment ratio of stage I NPC is 76.9%.

In the early stage it is very difficult to find out focuses in pharyngeal recess and pharyngeal base due to a covered nasopharyngeal position. Headache, nasal obstruction, nasal hemorrhage and tinnitus are usually misjudged as indisposition. Many patients with those symptoms will delay seeing a doctor. Many patients come to see a oculist because of strabismus, diplopic or hypopsia. Some patients casually take Chinese medicine or anodyne for their headache. Some patients who have enlargement of cervical lymph nodes were wrongly treated as TB or inflammation, thus delayed their treatment until the late stage of NPC.

If focus is located in deep layer of nasopharyngeal mucosa or pharyngeal recess, the patients may have no symptoms at all in the early stage. So the author suggests that the following should be carried out:

(1) The items of NPC in general health check-up should be carried out

In China's southeast coastline areas, such as Guangdong, Guangxi, Hunan, Fujian etc, where the NPC is popular, the necessary check-up items of NPC such as the serum VCA-IgA antibody should be carried out in the annual check-up.

Any patient whose VCA-IgA anti body with a positive titer>1:5 should undergo further check. For example, execute EBNA examination of nasopharynx smear and observe the exfoliative cells by microscope, take biopsy and check classification when necessary, in the hope of diagnosis and treatment as earlier as possible.

(2) Set up the anti-cancer out-patient service everywhere, launch the tumor census

The results of 480 000 people census in some regions of Guangdong province indicated that the ratio of stage I patients was 58.75%, which was 7.57 times of that (7.1%) in the out-patient service of the Tumor Hospital of Sun Yat-sen University. All the patients found by the census have ear-nose symptoms, but they did not attach importance to the symptoms and see a doctor. This shows that general survey can raise the cure rate by earlier diagnosis and treatment.

(3) Check in earnest and listen carefully to patients' chief complains during the examination

Make careful examination, check in earnest and induct the patients to tell their chief complains; in order to prevent patients from misregarding migraine, tinnitus and nasal hemorrhage etc. as unimportant illnesses. If the primary carcinoma is in the parietal wall of nasopharynx, the patients may have nasal obstruction and nasal hemorrhage, if the primary carcinoma is in the pharyngeal recess and the lateral wall of nasopharynx, the patients may often have tinnitus hypoacusis or otitis.

(4) Macrography features

At present, biopsy by pharyngorhinoscopy is very convenient and accurate. If fleck and rough surface can be seen by pharyngorhinoscopy, it must be squamous cells hyperplasia or squamous epithelia metaplasia from columnar epithelia; if dead gray or nodal nasopharyngeal mucosa can be seen, it must be apophysis under mucosa, invading, as well as erosive, ulcerating and bloody. In this condition, biopsy and histological classification should be done, and then accurate treatment projects made.

(5) Serological diagnosis of EB-virus

The difference of serum EB-virus antibody between NPC patients and normal persons is significant, so this item is an important check index; and it is very convenient for check-up and survey of tumor. The reaction of serum EB-virus antibody of NPC patients is characteristic of IgA-antibody rising. Henle[9] has reported that its positive ratio was 93%, and positive ratio of 1006 cases in the Tumor Hospital of Sun Yat-sen University was 93.83%(944 positive cases, antibody titer of $\geqslant$1:5). If taking antibody titer >1:10 as positive, there are 90.9% NPC patients.

The rising of VCA-IgA antibody level can be used to estimate patients' disease development; the antibody level of clinical stage-Ⅳ and N3 patients with cervical metastasis are higher 3~4 times than that of the clinical stage-I and N0 patients. Besides, positive VCA-IgA antibody is helpful for us to discover the unseen NPC that are located in the pharyngeal recess and under pharyngeal mucosa. It can also call the attention of doctors and patients to trace the primary focus within a short period so as to avoid delayed diagnosis.

Zeng Yi etc.[10] reported that the positive ratio of EBNA examination of exfoliative cell of nasopharyngeal smears was 100%. It is very helpful to diagnose invading NPC which is located under nasopharyngeal mucosa and with negative biopsy. EBNA antigen combined with VCA—IgA examination is very useful to diagnosis of NPC with negative biopsy.

(6) Radiograph and CT diagnosis of NPC

NPC diagnosis depended on clinical examination and biopsy, while Radiograph and CT check are assistant measures. In order to confirm the condition of basicranial bones, lungs, liver and other bones of the body and to see the sizes and ranges of local mass, the doctors may perform this examination. The bones involved may have osteolytic defect or enlargement of the normal foramen and canal with unclear and irregular edges. The bones are dissymmetric compared with the normal sides. Also it helps us to find out the relationship between skull bones with are destroyed and the symptoms of cranial nerves invaded, such as headache, diplopic, blurred vision and facial anesthesia.

Radiograph shows bone absorption of cervical foramen, unclear edges, enlargement of normal foramen, and that both sides are dissymmetric. In particular, for some cases that cannot be observed by pharyngorhinoscopy, barium plaster contrast Radiograph examination should be carried out to find the smaller primary focus. For example, Radiograph shows one side of pharyngeal recess shoaling, disappearing or moving forward; both sides are dissymmetric, one side of pharyngeal carina is incrassated, swelling or shortening. The nozzle is striated, the posterior wall of nasopharynx is incrassated and rugged as well as local apophysis under postterior wall. In this condition, biopsy by pharyngorhinoscopy or cytology of nasopharynx is necessary to draw up accurate treatment projects.

4. Differential diagnosis of nasopharyngeal carcinoma (NPC), other benign and malignant tumors of nasus,nasopharynx and tumor-like, inflammatory diseases

Since the treatment projects and prognosis of NPC, other benign and malignant tumors of nasus, nsopharynx and tumor-like, inflammatory diseases are completely different, it is essential for the doctors to oserve the patients carefully by pharyngorhinoscopy, combined with biopsy and puncture, when possible, to make pathological diagnosis. Histochemical and immunohistochemcal examination should be taken if necessary.

4.1 Chronic hyperplasic inflammation of nasopharynx(Fig.28–30)

Nasal obstruction is common. Nasal hemorrhage and tinnitus are rare. If inflammatory and plump mucosa of nasopharynx obstructs auditory tubal prominence, the patients may have tinnitus, which is always temporary and may disappear after the inflammation fades away. Pharyngorhinoscopy shows diffusely granular, rugged and wet mucosa, microscopy shows lymph follicle of nodular hyperplasia, plump parts without obvious border. If anything is in doubt, biopsy and cytological smear should be taken.

4.2 Hyperplastic tuberculosis of nasopharyngeal mucosa(Fig.31, 32)

Tuberculosis may cause incrassation of nasopharyngeal mucosa, local nasal obstruction or pyoid and bloody snot. Pharyngorhinoscopy shows irregular ulcerous borderline and having cheesy secretion on its surface. Smear shows necrotic materials without carcinoma cells. Microscopy shows tuberculosis focus made up of epithelial cells and Langhan's giant cells with horseshoe multinucleus.

4.3 Fungal nasopharyngitis(Fig.35–42)

This atlas collects refractory hyperplastic chronic rhinitis and nasopharyngitis resulting from fungal infection,such as actinomycosis,moniliasis, etc. Nasopharyngitis may cause nasopharyngeal epithelia hyperplasia or atypical hyperplasia. Cytological smear shows heteromorphic cells. It is necessary to do biopsy and fungal culture for diagnosis.

4.4 Coccidioidomyocosis (coccidioidal granuloma) of nasus and North American blastomycosis (Fig.183–185)

This is also one of the nasal inflammations of fungal infection. Tumor-like neoplasm may appear and spread to the nasopharynx. The patients may have a long course of disease with ulcer, pyoid and bloody snot. If erotion and ulcer occur, fungal culture of secretion and biopsy is helpful for diagnosis and antifungal therapy is efficient.

4.5 Leprosy of nasus(Fig.174–182)

Leprosy of nasus also spreads from nasus to nasopharynx, and nasopharyngeal mucosa incrassation, nodular hyperplasia or ulceration may occur. The patients may have a long course of disease with nasal obstruction, but lack of headache, tinnitus and cranial nerve symptoms. If no symptoms of body skin appear, biopsy and acid-fast staining are necessary for diagnosis.

4.6 lymphoma of nasopharynx(Fig.140–159)

Lymphoma of nasopharynx are the second most common malignant tumors of nasopharynx, next to NPC. The results of the analysis of 121 cases of nasopharyngeal lymphoma in the tumor hospital of Sun Yat-sen University indicated that NHL (non-Hodgkin's Lymphoma) was 84.3%, while HD (Hodgkin's disease) was 15.7%. Pharyngorhinoscopy showed that the type of plump mass accounted for 60.7%, and nodular type for 25.5% [11]. Ulceration was rare. The surface was gray-reddish and wet; the texture was solid, and enlargement of cervical lymph nodes was common. Knubbly cervical lymph nodes were more active than those with carcinoma metastasis. Cranial nerves were not involved.

The Most likely differential diagnosis depended on biopsy and pathological diagnosis. Microscopy showed that the tumor was made up of diffuse and round lymphocytes. Immunohistochemical LCA antibody was significant for diagnosis. The treatment project of Lymphoma of nasopharynx is totally different from that of NPC. Chemotherapy has the priority.

4.7 Benign tumor of nasopharygeal mesenchyma (Fig.118–131)

Although hemangioma of nasopharynx may cause nasal hemorrhage, the blood is cardinal red and hemorrhage is more severe. Pharyngorhinoscopy shows that red and soft mass heaves towards the nasopyaryngeal mucosa. If neoplasm near postnaris, the patient may have nasal obstruction. The pathological changes develop slowly, and the patient may have a long course of disease, without Lymph node metastasis. In addition, both neurofibroma and leiomyoma of nasopharynx are benign tumors, with solid texture, slow development and clear borderline. They can be resected by surgery and diagnosed by biopsy.

4.8 Malignant tumor of nasopharygeal mesenchyma (Fig.132–139)

Rhaodomyosarcoma, leiomyosarcoma and chordoma of nasopharynx are rare malignant tumors of nasopharynx. It grows fast, with soft texture, erosion and necrosis, infection. The patient may have hemorrhage or pyoid or bloody snot. Differential diagnosis is based mostly on pathological morphology, histochemistry and immunohistochemistry.

5. Some Problems concerning misdiagnosis of NPC

5.1 Both doctors and patients do not pay adequate attention to early diagnosis because primary focus of NPC is secluded

Primary focus is located in nasopharynx, with slight early symptoms and without general discomfort such as nasal obstruction, nasal himmorhage or bloody tinged snot. Tinnitus and headache happen occationally. Patients do not go to see a doctor until knubbly lymph nodes appear in the neck or they have conscious strabismus, diplopia of or severe hemocrania, at the moderate or late stage of the illness. This is the main cause of low cure ratio.

5.2 Medical market competition

Patients may be treated by heteropathy in general clinics so they do not go to see a doctor in specialized hospital in time. There are no whole set of equipments and technique of nasopharyngeal check-up in general clinics. Thus the patients do not reveived necessary examination of nasopharyngeal carcinoma and the diagnosis may be delayed.

5.3 Importance is not attached to EB-virus related examination.

Doctors in general clinics do not attach importance to examination of serous VCA-IgA antibody level. Of the 1006 NPC cases of the Tumor Hospital of Sun Yat-sen University, 93.8% of the patients´serum VCA-IgA antibody levels were positive and their titers were all beyond 1:5 ~1:10, with the tiptop reaching 1:1280. We therefore suggest that all persons of general health checkup and all patients of E.N.T. department should received the examination of serous VCA-IgA antibody level. And any patient with serous titer beyond 1:5 and focus not found by examination of nasopharynx should be reexamined periodically.

5.4 Misdiagnosis of enlargement of jugular lymph nodes for inflammation and tuberculosis

Many patients came to the Tumor Hospital of Sun Yat-sen University after they had been treated inefficiently by anti-inflammatory and anti-tuberculous therapy at other hospitals. Some patients did not come to doctor until their lymph nodes of neck enlarged because the tumor invading submucosa, or the tumor was located in auditory tube, and which was not found by pharyngorhinoscopy, 45.3% of the 1000 patients of tumor hospital of Sun Yat-sen University had enlargement of jugular lymph node as primary symptom. While 10.65% of them had enlargement of jugular lymph nodes as unique symptom. Most of these patients were in moderate stage of the illness. Serum VCA-IgA antibody examination or EBNA by cervical lymph nodes puncture biopsy should be carried out immediately. If both are positive, pathological biopsy should be done for diagosis.

5.5 The misplay of clinical work

Although patients have nasal obstruction, nasal hemorrhage, tinnitus and otalgia, or their tumor focus cant's be seen clearly by pharyngorhinoscopy, with many times negative biopsies, some patients do not come to consult a doctor about their condition. They come to see a doctor only when the lymph node has metastasized or involved cranial nerves.

5.6 Misplay of pathological work

Diagnosis cannot be made because check-lists are too simple, symptoms of NPC and conditions seen by pharyngorhinoscopy are not provided or the tissue of biopsy is too small or heavy jamming. Some positive patients are misdiagnosed as negative ones due to unstandardized technique or because the biopsy sample of benign nasopharyngeal nodes misses the malignant tissue, leading to the delay treatment of the positive patients. Patients with nasopharyngeal nodes are not sensitive to radiation therapy, on the contrary they may suffer from radition injury and economic loss.

6. Some problems about treatment of NPC

This atlas emphasizes histomorphological types and related diagnosis of NPC. William etc.[12] reviewed 177 papers on treatment, none of them touched upon the morphological classification; most of them phasized radiotherapy and chemotherapy. A few of these papers referred to treatment development of EB-virus gene therapy and biological, immune therapy. Fee We Jr. [13] indicated that for patients who had palatal fistula, trismus or residual focus after radical radiotherapy, selective surgery would have satisfafctory long-term results. The 5-year actuarial control rate of tumors in nasopyarynx is about 65%, while the 5-year disease-free survival rate is around 54%. The authors shows that if patients have well differentiated squamous cell carcinoma or adenocarcinoma of NPC, as well as those who are insensitive to radiotherapy and chemo-therapy, their tumors should be removed adequately on early stage, combined with immune therapy plus EB gene therapy and the results will be satisfactory. For example, Mr. Gan, an apothecary, at the age of 60 had recurrent tumors seven years after treatment of NPC. His biopsy showed nasopharyngeal carcinoma in situ, and his total nasopharyngeal mucosa was removed adequately; his pathological diagnosis was polycentric nasopharyngeal carcinoma in situ. He still survives well after a 10-year follow-up. (A man, 45 years old, had nasopharyngeal adenoid cystic carcinoma. Radiotherapy had no effect on him the focus did not disappear, and the stromal had malignant fibro histocytoma Fig.113–116.) If the patient could have his carcinoma removed adequately at early stage and combined with gene therapy and immune therapy, the results would have been satisfactory.

7 References

1. 梁伯强, 祝家镇. 鼻咽癌组织发生学的研究 I. 全部鼻咽的新解剖法及鼻咽粘膜的一般形态改变. 中华病理学杂志, 1960.6: 257
2. 梁伯强著. 鼻咽癌的组织学类型, 生物学特性和组织发生学的研究. 上海科学技术出版社. 1962,7: 15
3. Leon Barnes, Jone W. Eveson, Peter Reichard, et al. World health organization classification of tumours. Pathology&Genetice of Head neck tumours. (IARC press lyon 2005)
4. 中山医学院肿瘤研究所病理免疫研究室著. 鼻咽部癌变过程的形态发生学(初步研究). 新医学 (肿瘤研究专辑), 1975,11:1.
5. 陈剑经. 鼻咽粘膜上皮癌变过程形态学进一步研究. 中山医学院肿瘤研究所学术资料选编(一). 肿瘤病理研究, 1976,48–53.
6. 李振权,潘启超,陈剑经等. 鼻咽癌临床与实验研究. 广东科学技术出版社, 1983,199–208
7. Chen–yulin. Lympho-epithelioma of the Nasopharynx with involvement of the nervous system. Chin Med J, 1985, 98: 1075
8. 梁伯强,陈剑经,祝家镇等. 广东鼻咽癌组织学类型生物学特性和组织发生学的研究. 中华医学杂志, 1962,81:629
9. Henle G;Epstein-Barr virus-specific IgA serum antibodies as an out standing feature of nasopharyngeal carcinoma. Int J Cancer, 1976, 17: 1–7
10. 曾毅, 皮国华,赵文平. 检查 EB 病毒核抗原的补体免疫酶法的建立. 中国医学科学院学报, 1980, 2:134–135
11. Lu Xianyu, Wu Qiuliang. Clinicopathologic Analysis On 121 Cases of Nasal and Nasopharyngeal Lymphoma (NPL). Chin J Cancer Res, 1993,5:205–210.
12. William I Wei, Jonathan S T Sham. Nasopharyngeal carcinoma. Lancet, 2005,365:2041–2050
13. Fee WE Jr, Moir MS, Choi EC, et al. Nasopharyngectomy for recurrent nsopharyngeal carcer: a2 –to 17 –year follow –up. Arch Otolaryngol Head Neck Surg, 2002,128:280–284

2 Pathology atlas

1. Gross findings of nasopharyngeal carcinoma (NPC) and other nasopharyngeal diseases:

Gross appearance

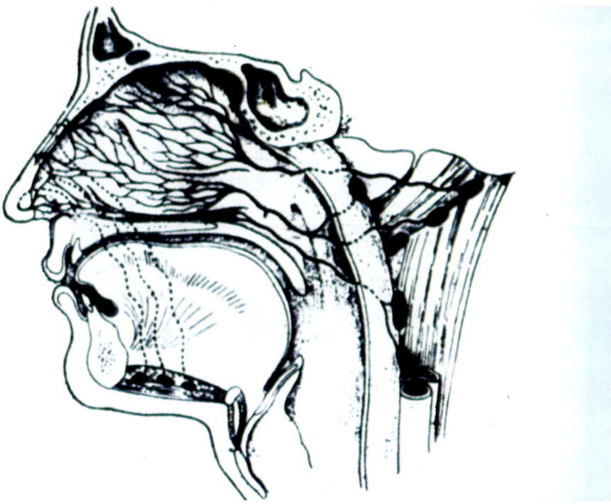

Fig.1 Lateal section of nose, nasopharynx and oral cavity (lateral view)

Figure 1 showed the communication between nose and nasopharyn and the distribution of cervical lymph nodes in order to realizing the common metastatic pathway of NPC to cervical lymph nodes.

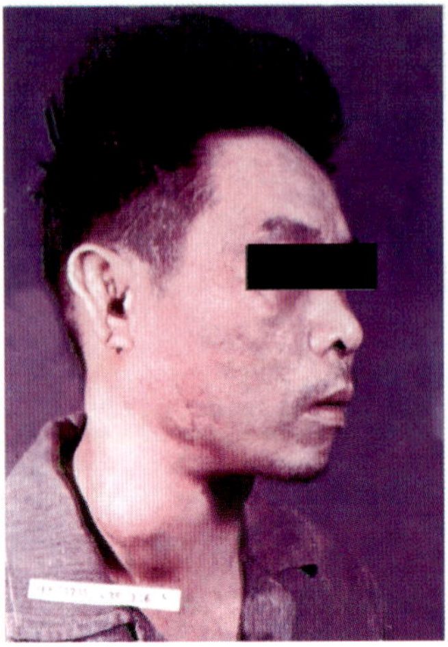

Fig.2 NPC with metastasis tumor in neck (lateral view)

Male, 48 years old. NPC, clinic stage III, had a lump at neck for one year more, no nasal obstruction, nasal hemorrhage and headache. Pathological diagnosis showed Squamous cell carcinoma (grade III) of nasopharynx.

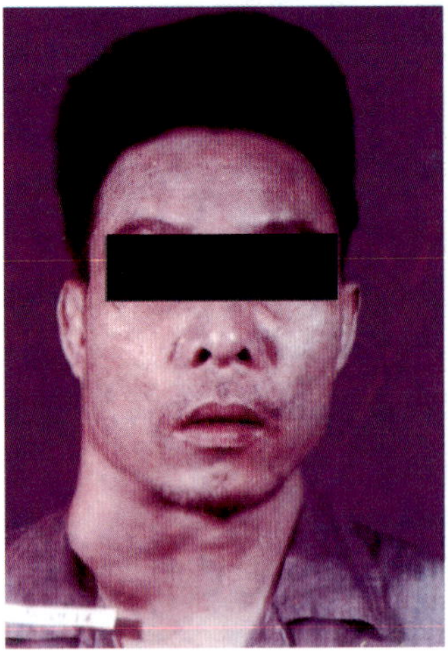

Fig.3 NPC with metastatic tumor mass in neck (front view, same case as in Fig.2)

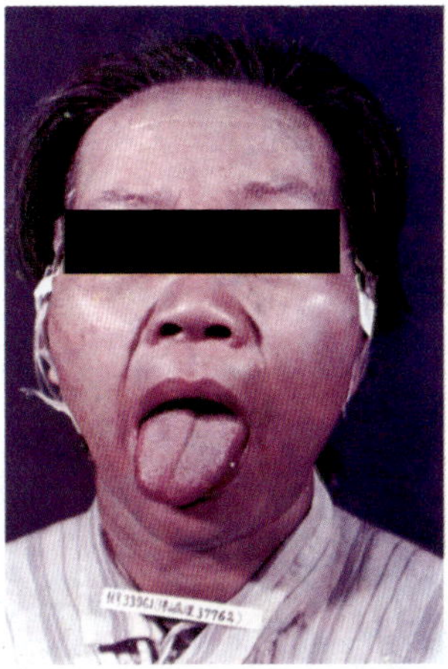

Fig.4 Cranial nerves involved by NPC

Female, 51 years old, base of the skull and right hypoglossal nerve were invaded by NPC, inducing a right deviation of tongue during stretching out from the mouth.

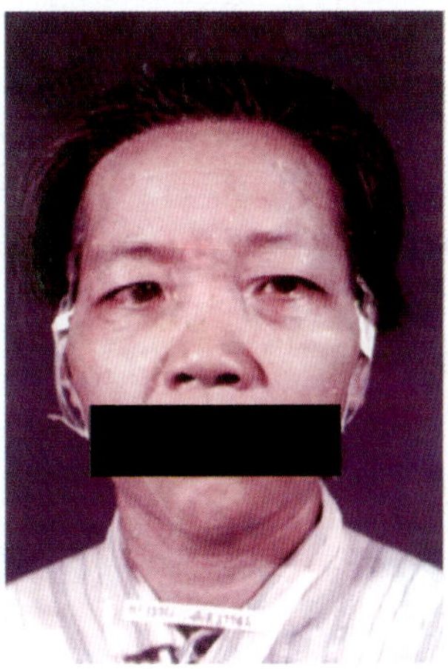

Fig.5 Cranial nerves involved by NPC
(same as Fig.4 Involved abducent nerve)

Patient's abducent nerve was involved by NPC causing convergent strabismus of the eyes. Patient had also symptom of diplopia.

From Fig. 6–15: Gross appearance of whole portion of nasopharynx tissue separated and removed along Liang–zhu's technique for autopsy of NPC patients (addendum 1)

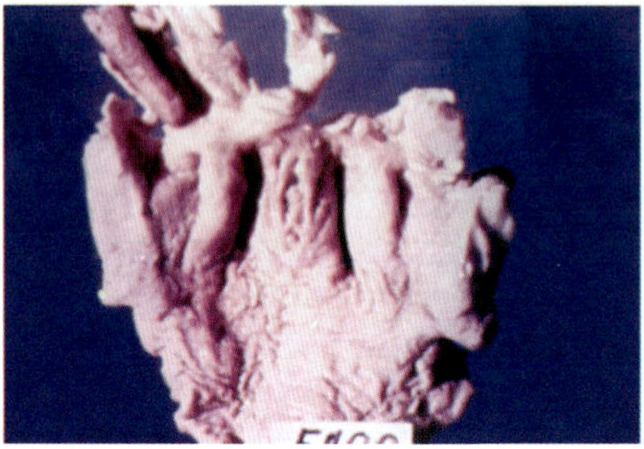

Fig.6 Chronic inflammation of nasopharyngeal mucosa (Macroscopic image)

Male, 58 years old. The nasopharyngeal mucosa became thickened and rough by chronic inflammation, the pharyngeal tonsils locating between the Rosen–Műller's fossi, also became thickened and cord–like in appearance.

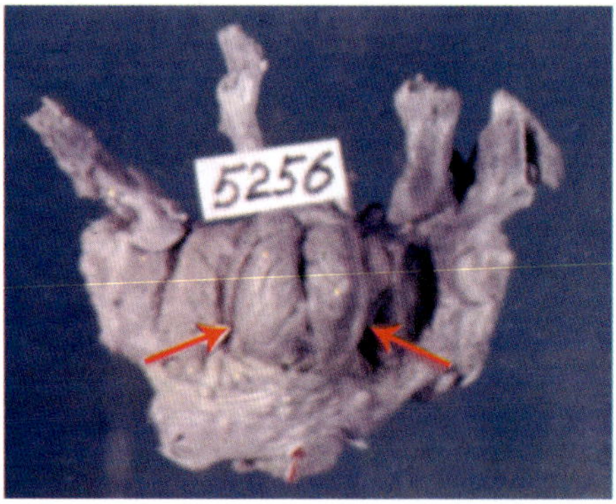

Fig.7 Tumor–like hyperplasia of nasopharyngeal lymph tissue

Female, 25 years old, chronic inflammation of nasopharyngeal mucosa, Pharyngeal tonsils proliferated, nodular in appearance, protruding above the surface, with small proliferative follicles along the peripheral margin, which microscopically, were the proliferaative lymph follicles. This lesion is known as adenoid clinically.

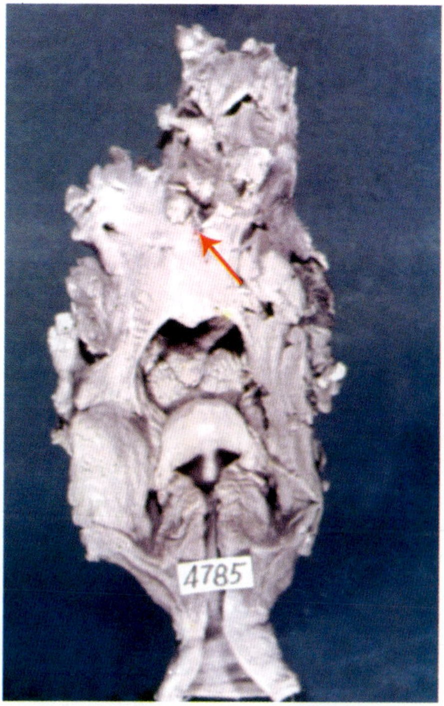

Fig.8 Nodular type NPC

Male, 43 years old, had a lump in right neck for four years more, pathological diagnosis of biopsy tissue was: squamous cell carcinoma (grade III) with metastasis in rignt neck. Patient had not received any specific treatment. He developed nasal hemorrhage and ordorous nasal discharge one year before the admission and the metaststic lump in neck became larger gradually. Patient finally developed severe headache and died of cachexia.

Figure showed the whole portion of nasopharynx separated and removed during autopsy, including soft palate, larynx and trachea. Grossly a nodular NPC was obtained at the right posterior part of parietal lateral-wall of nasopharynx (arrow), with infiltration to right nasal conchae and posterior nares. Metastatic focuses of NPC were seen in cervical lymph nodes bilaterally and right side supraclavicular lymph nodes. Some metastatic cervical lymph nodes were perforated and tumor cell thrombi found in jugular vein. There were also metastatic foci seen in thoracic vertebrae, left ileum, left maxilla, and right temporal lobe plus dura mater of the brain.

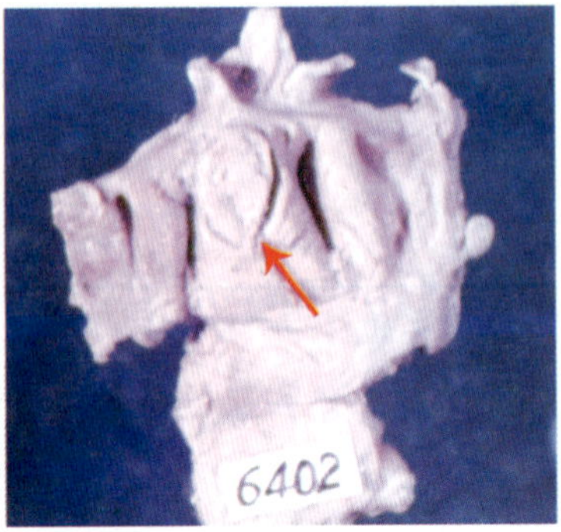

Fig.9 Nodular type NPC

Female, 24 years old, had right nasal obstruction and headache for two more years, followed by hypopsia, diplopia and facial paralysis. After radiotherapy, she developed myeloativemalacia, then hand-foot paresis, numbness of the trunk and fially died of respiratory paralysis.

Arrow showed nodular focus of NPC. Pathological diagnosis by biopsy was Pleomorphic cell carcinoma of nasopharynx.

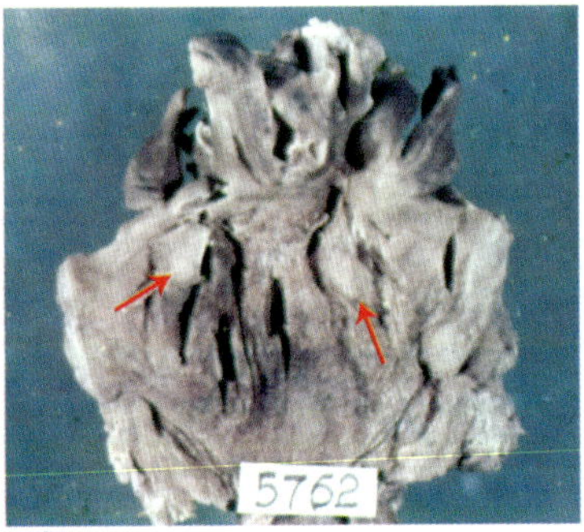

Fig.10 NPC, ulcerous type

Male, 62 years old, had a history of lumps in neck bilaterally for 1 year more, usually accompanying with nasal obstruction and nasal hemorrhage, and later on short breathing developed.

Two arrows showed the range of the ulcer. The ulcer base was uneven. A metastatic focus at left soft palate was $0.5\times0.5\times0.4cm^3$ in size. There were metaststsis in cervical lymph nodes of both sides, lymph nodes of supraclavicular region and anterior mediastinum, as well as the right cervical sympathetic ganglia. Tumor cell thrombi were obtained in right jugular vein.

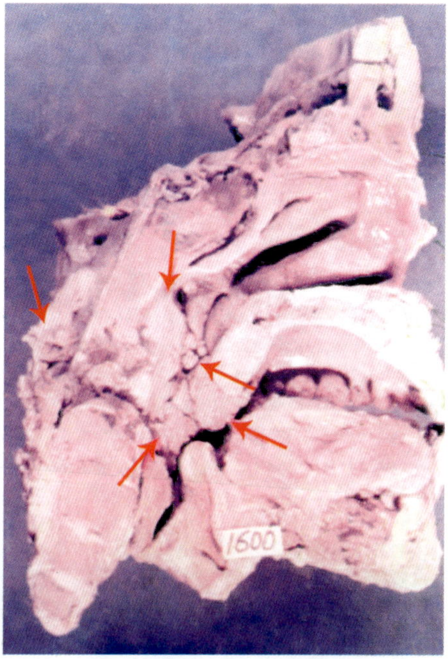

Fig.11 NPC, Cauliflower type

Male, 33 years old, besides nasal obstruction, tinnitus, deaf, nasal hemorrhage, bloody sputum, halitosis, left jugular lumps patient had also dyspnea, dysphagia and finally died of multiple organ failure.

Arrow showed the invasive area of NPC. The tumor extended from the parietal wall towards the posterior wall of nasopharynx, then to the pharynx, soft palate, posterior nares, and down towards to the esophagus orifice. The tumor mass protruded from the mucosa surface, cauliflower in appearance. Invasion of base of the skull, the sphenoidal sinus, cervical vertebrae, and soft palate by NPC could be seen grossly at autopsy. There were generalized lymph node metastasis including lungs, liver, spleen, pericardium and the posterior lobe of pituitary gland.

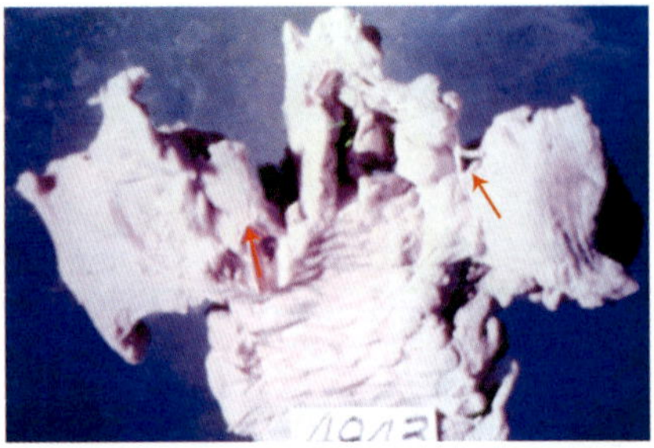

Fig.12 Nodular type NPC

Female, 29 years old, had tinnitus, hypoacusis, dizziness, pain of anterior chest region, and wandering pain over chest and back for three months.

Arrows had pointed out a nodule at the of right parietal wall of nasopharynx, $0.5cm\times0.4cm\times0.3cm^3$ in size. The tumor extended from the original site to the sphenoidal bone. There were metastasis in cervical and supraclavicular lymph nodes, multiple ribs, sternum, right humerus, vertebrae and liver.

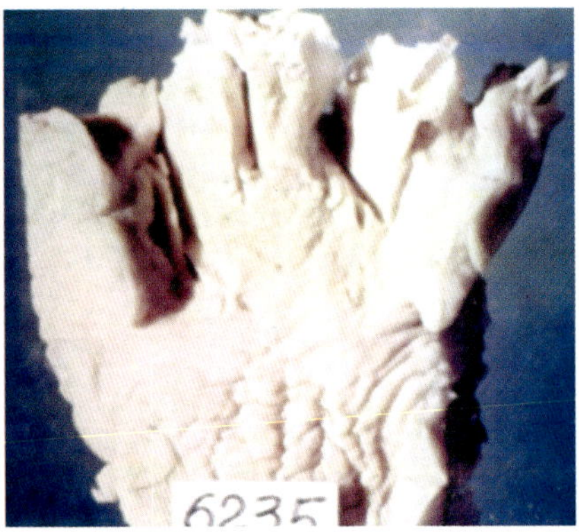

Fig.13 NPC after radiotherapy
(gross finding, the primary carcinoma had vanished)

Female, 16 years old, with a pathological diagnosis by biopsy of spindle cell carcinoma (Non keratinizing carcinoma)of nasopharynx. Eight months after radiotherapy,she felt pain over the inguinal regions in both sides and later on, pain of lumber vertebrae. Patient finaly passed away by cachexia. Autopsy evealed metastasis focuses in lymph glands of inguinal region, peripancreatic, and portal areas, liver, cervical and lumbar vertebrae, however, the primary cancer focus was not found.

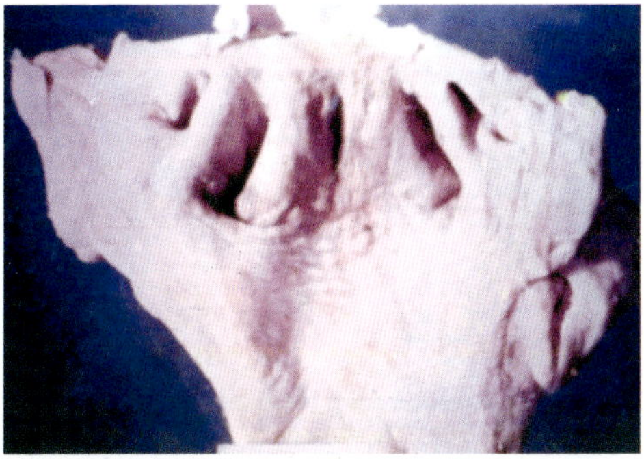

Fig.14 Atrophy of nasopharyngeal mucosa

Male, 49 years old. Figure showed a smooth nasopharyngeal mucosa, lymph follicles not distinguishable.

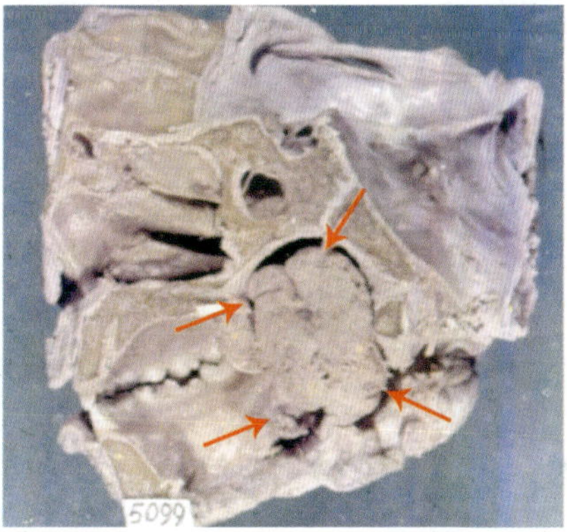

Fig.15 Non-Hodgkin lymphoma of nasopharynx

Male, 9 years old, had asaphia for 32 days. Patient felt also obstructive sensation accompanied with purulent and bloody sputum, emaciation and finally died of high fever and infection.

Arrows showed that patient's oral, nasal and pharyngeal cavities were filled up by a solid tumor mass, grey-reddish in color. The posterior nares, larynx and opening of esophagus were nearly completely blocked by the tumor mass. Autopsy revealed diffused metastasis in organs of different cavities including pericardium, both side kidneys and adrenals, pancreas, liver with partial capsule, duodenum, greater omentum, deep cervical lymph nodes left, cervical sympathetic ganglia and posterior peritoneal wall of the abdominal cavity.

2. Pharyngorhinoscopy

Fig.16 –27: Gross appearance of different types of NPC by pharyngorhinoscopy.

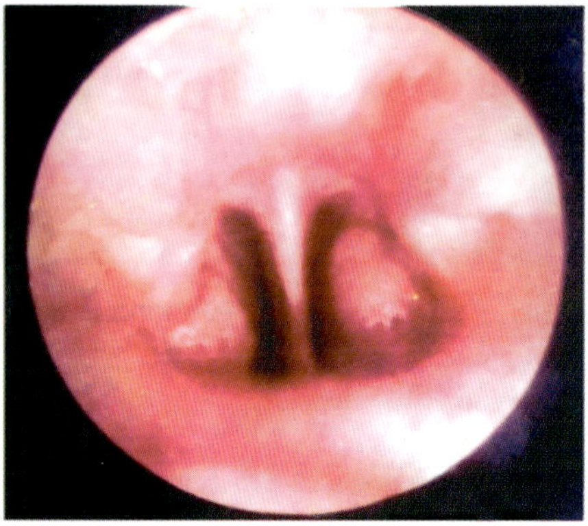

Fig.16 Adenoid proliferation of nasopharyngeal mucosa

The nasopharyngeal mucosa was relatively intact. There was benign hypertrophy of adenoid at the posterior parietal wall of nasopharynx. Posterior nares became narrow in both sides. Patient had nasal obstruction, but without symptom and signs of NPC including nasal hemorrhage, tinnitus, and headache etc..

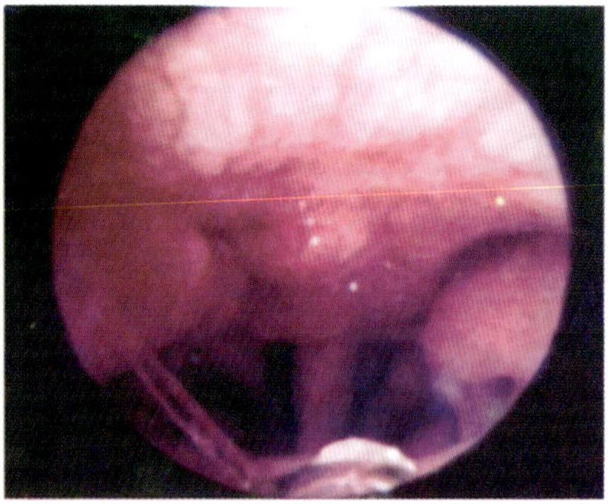

Fig.17 Nodular type NPC

Male, 40 years old. Pharyngorhinoscopy showed nodular protrusion of the primary focus of NPC.

Clinical stage: $T_1N_2M_0$

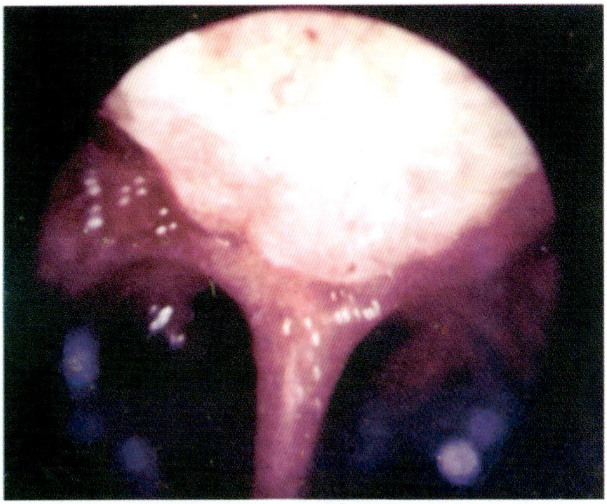

Fig.18 Nodular type NPC

Male, 52 years old. Pharyngorhinoscopy showed a large nodule locating at the posterior parietal wall of nasopharynx. Pharyngeal recess disappeared.

Clinical stage: $T_4N_3M_0$

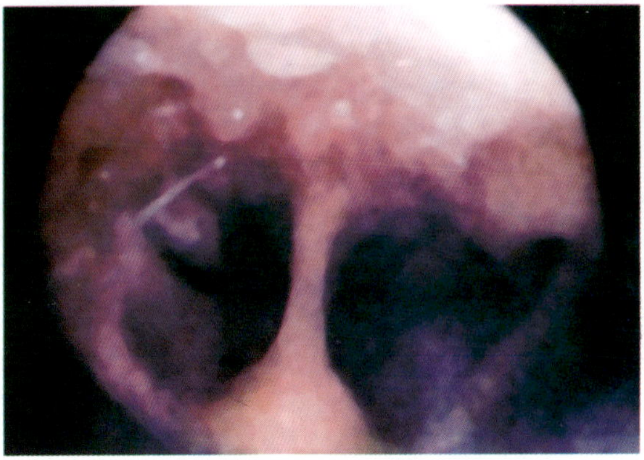

Fig.19 Infiltrative type NPC

Male, 36 years old. Pharyngorhinoscopy showed that the parietal lateral wall of nasopharynx was invaded by a neoplasm. The surface became rough and uneven and tumor's margin unclear. Both pharyngeal recess and orifices of Eustachian tubes were difficult to be identified.

Clinical stage: $T_2N_0M_0$

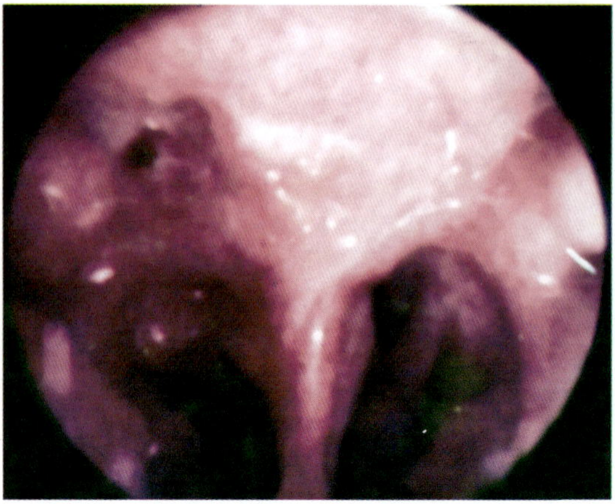

Fig.20　Infiltrative type NPC

Male, 33 years old. Pharyngorhinoscopy showed the neoplasm locating at the upper portin of the posterior parietal wall in both sides and infiltrated along the lateral wall of nasopharynx. Ulceration was seen in one of the tumor growths.

Clinical stage: T_3N_2M0

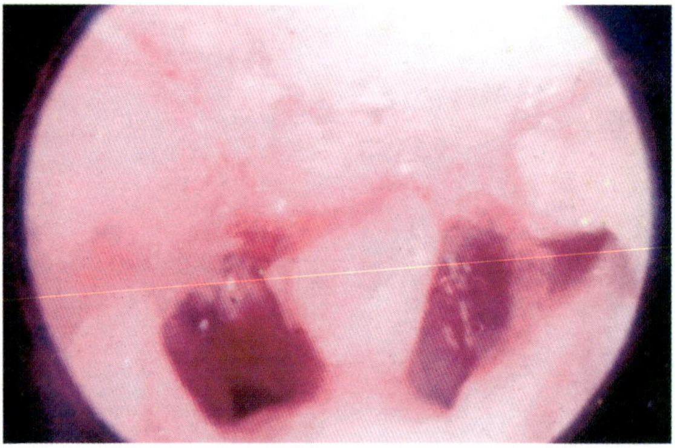

Fig.21　Ulcerous and Infiltrative type NPC

Female, 44 years old. Pharyngorhinoscopy showed infiltration of carcinoma cells in the prietal part and both lateral walls of the nasopharynx as well as the posterior nares, causing deformity of orifices of both naises. Both pharyngeal recess and orifices of the Eustachian tubes were also not visible.

Clinical stage:$T_3N_0M_0$

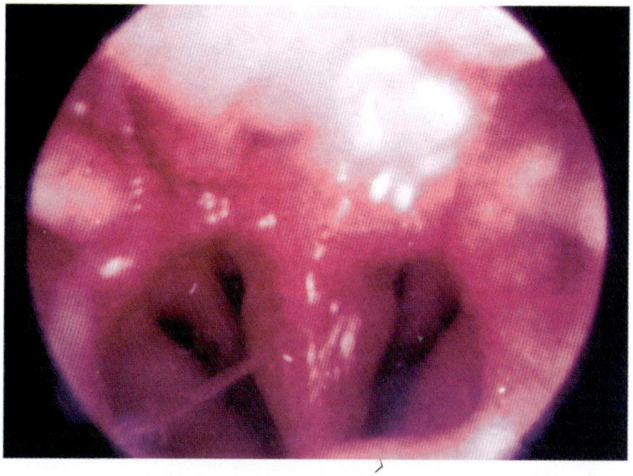

Fig.22 Infiltrative type NPC

Male, 47 years old. Pharyngorhinoscopy showed that the parietal wall and both lateral walls of nasopharynx were invaded by carcinoma cells, the lining mucosa became rough and even, both sides posterior nares unsymmetrical and one of them became narrowed.

Clinical stage: $T_3N_2M_0$

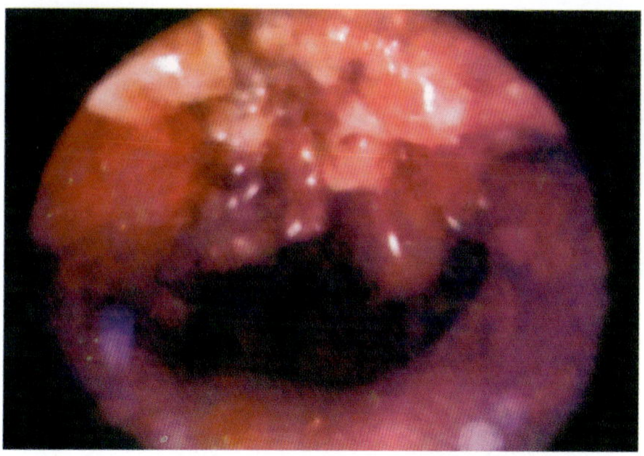

Fig.23 Cauliflower type NPC

Male, 45 years old. Pharyngorhinoscopy showed a cauliflower-like tumaor growth protruding at the parietal wall of nasopharynx and extended towards the posterior nares and both sides of the lateral walls. The pharyngeal recess and orifices of the Eustachian tubes were not identified.

Clinical stage: $T_3N_2M_0$

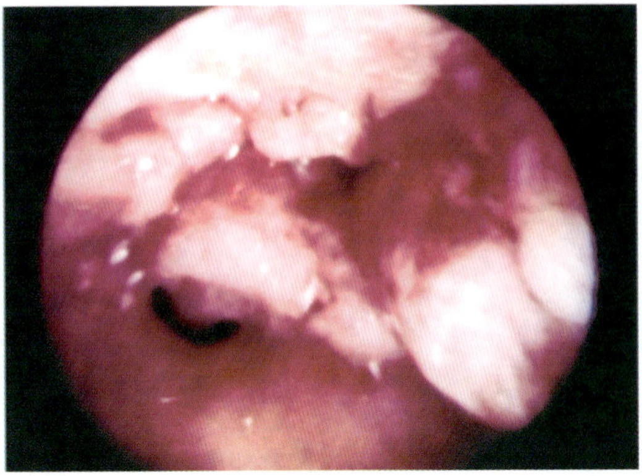

Fig.24　Cauliflower type NPC

Male, 46 years old. Pharyngorhinoscopy showed the tumor mass protruding from the parietal and lateral walls of nasopharynx, cauliflower in appearance with invasion to pharyngeal recess, Eustachian tubes and the posterior nares. There was ulceration of the tumor mass with exfoliation of the necrotic tissue. The posterior nares was obstructed by the tumor growth.

Clinical stage: $T_3N_2M_0$

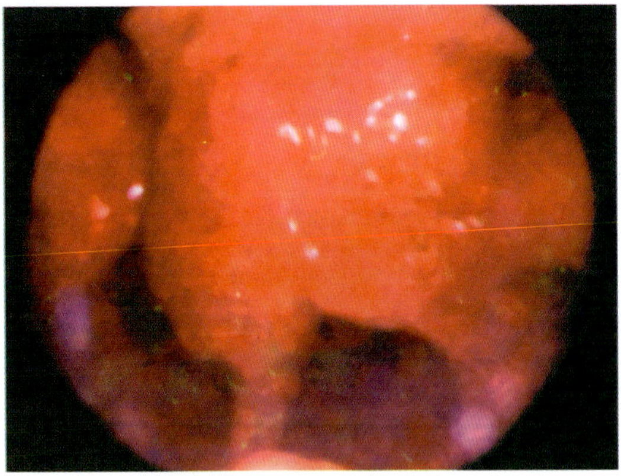

Fig.25　Bulky type NPC

Female, 33 years old. Pharyngorhinoscopy showed the neoplasm protruding from the parietal wall of nasopharynx and extended towards the posterior and both lateral walls.There was deformity of posterior nares.

Clinical stage: $T_3N_1M_0$

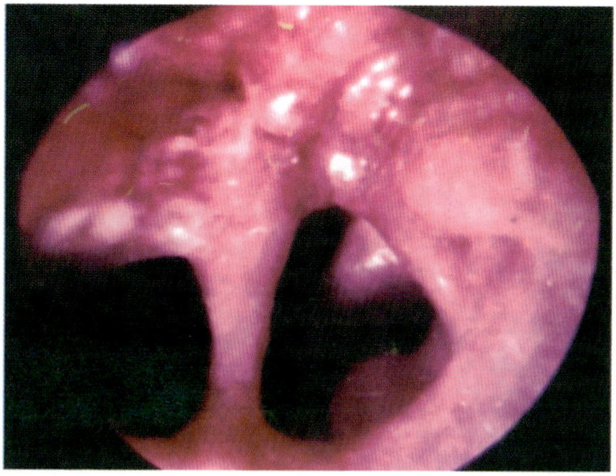

Fig.26 Ulcerative type NPC

Male, 42 years old. Pharyngorhinoscopy showed two ulcers locating on the parietal-lateral walls of both sides respectively. The border of ulcers became elevated and uneven, looking like a geographic map. The posterior nares were unsymmetrical.

Clinical stage: $T_3N_2M_0$

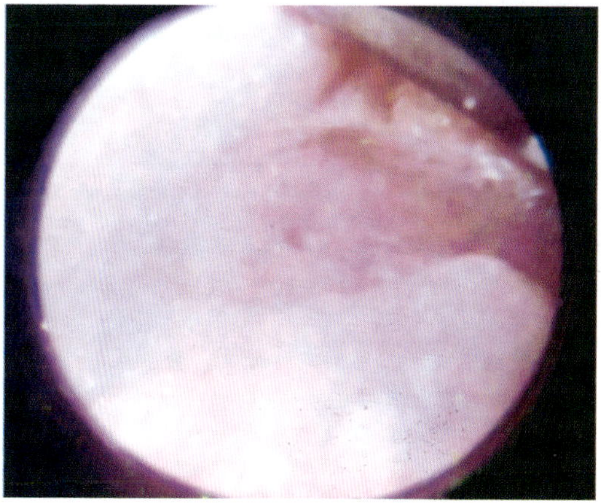

Fig.27 Diffused Infiltrating type NPC

Pharyngorhinoscopy showed a diffusely infiltration of carcinoma cells invading the posterior parietal wall and the lateral walls bilaterally of the nasopharynx and extended further towards the posterior nares.. The posterior nares and pharyngeal recess were unable to be identified.

Clinical stage: $T_3N_2M_0$

3. Histopatnological features of NPC and other diseases in nasopharynx

From Fig.28–170 were the histopathological changes of diseases of nasopharynx with special reference to different histopathological types of nasopharyngeal carcinoma (NPC)

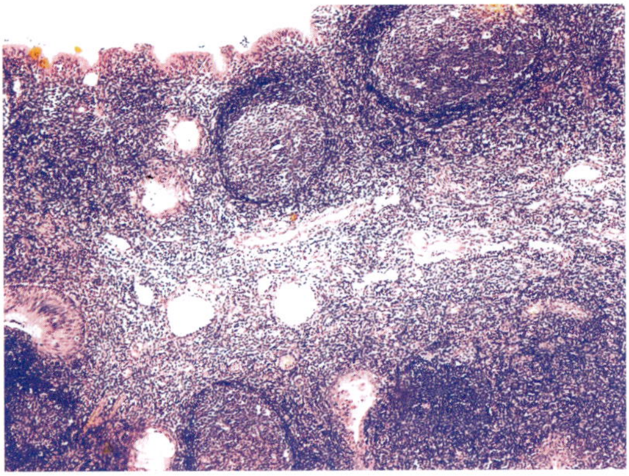

Fig.28 Chronic inflammation of nasopharynx mucosa

Male, 45 years old. Figure showed the mucosa surface to be covered by pseudostratified ciliated columnar epithelium, with massive lymphocytes infiltration under the epithelium and hyperplasia and hyperptrophy of the lmph folicles.(10×10)

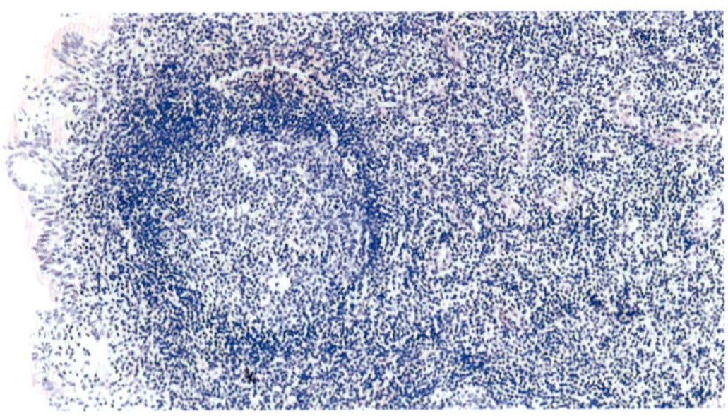

Fig.29 Chronic inflammation of nasopharynx mucosa (lymph follicles proliferative type)

Female, 25 years old. Pharyngorhinoscopy showed the nasopharyngeal mucosa to be granular in appearance due to mainly the proliferation of giant lymph follicles. (10×10)

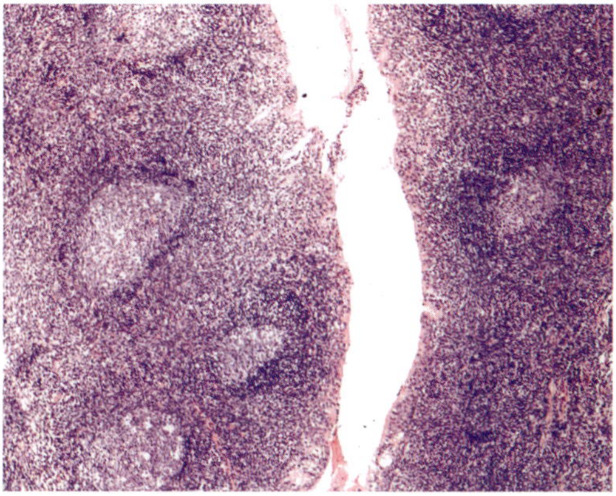

Fig.30 Chronic inflammation of nasopharynx mucosa (Same patient as in Fig.29, 10×10)

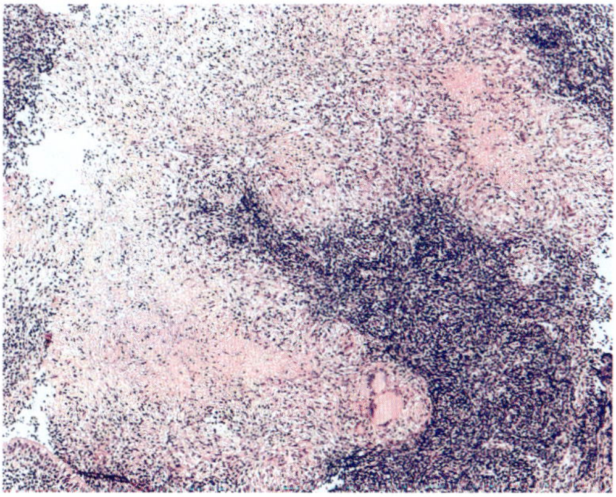

Fig.31 Proliferative type tuberculosis of nasopharynx

Female, 31 years old. Grossly, there was thickening of nasopharyngeal mucosa accompanied with localized ulceration. Microscopically, there were multiple tuberculous foci under the lamina propria, consisting of epithelioid cells, Langhan's giant cells and caseation . (10×10)

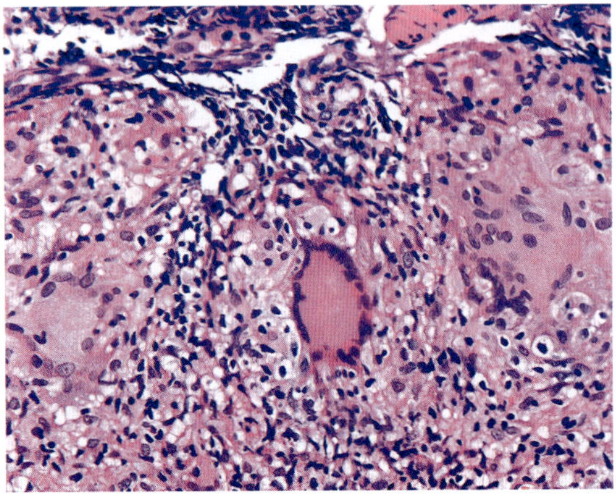

Fig.32 Proliferative type tuberculosis of nasopharynx (same patient as in Fig.31)

Figure 32 showed a typical Langerhans' cells, with plentiful cytoplasm and several tens nuclei which were horseshoe like in arrangement along the inner margin of the cell. (10×40)

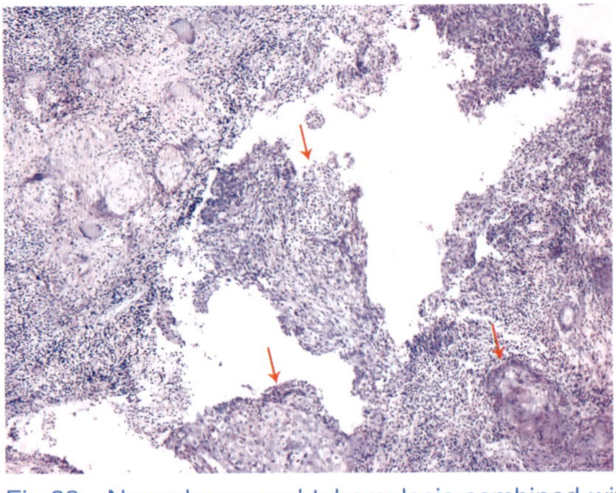

Fig.33 Nasopharyngeal tuberculosis combined with Poorly differentiated squamous cell carcinoma

Male, adult Figure showed two groups of irregular and poorly differentiated squamous cell carcinoma cell-nests (pointed by arrows) locating near by the tuberculous granulation tissue. (10×10)

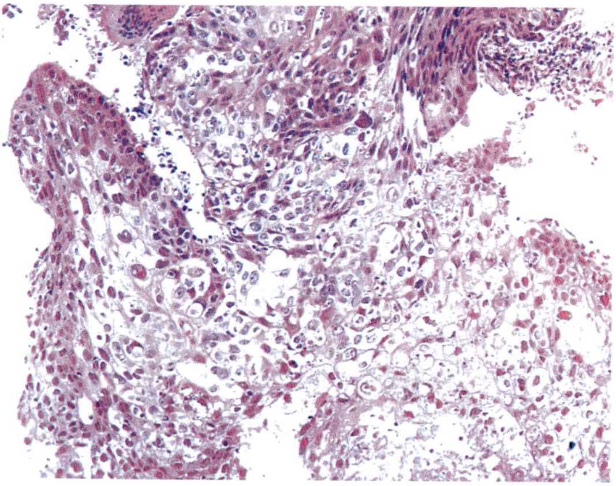

Fig.34 Nasopharyngeal tuberculosis combined with poorly-differentiated sauamous cell carcinoma (enlarged one of the 2 cancer cell nests showed in Fig.33,)

Figure showed the cancer cell-nest composing of oval and polygonal cells, pleomorphic and variation in size. Nuclei large, pleomorphic, mitotic figures occasionally can be seen. (10×40)

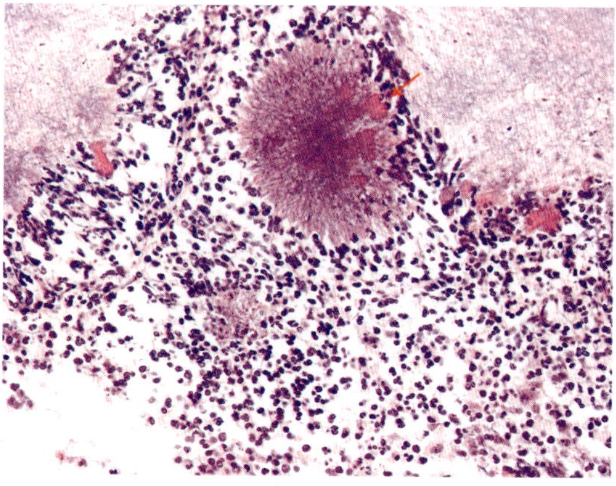

Fig.35 Chronic nasopharyngitis by Actinomycosis infection

Male, 42 years old. Figure showed the fungal clusters and sulfur granules which were surrounded by a large amount of neutrophils and mononuclear cells. (10×40)

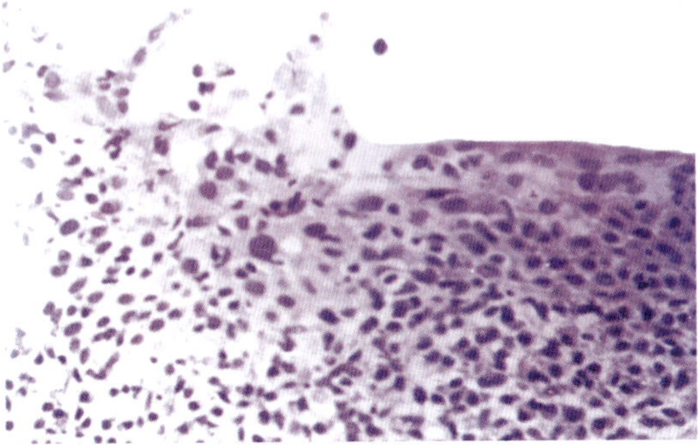

Fig.36 Actinomycosis infection of nasopharynx complicated with atypical hyperplasia of nasopharygeal mucosa (same case as in Fig. 35 , another field)

Figure showed atypical hyperplasia of the lining epithelial cells, nuclei enlarged, varying in size and hyperchromatic. The basement membrane was not intact with a tendency of malignant change.(10×40)

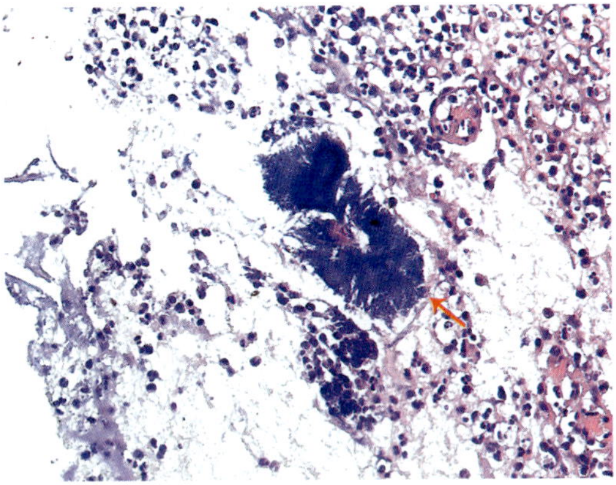

Fig.37 Fungal nasopharyngitis

Female, 34 years old. Figure 37 showed fungal clusters present in the necrotic and inflammatory exudate, morphologically like Aspergillosis infection accompaning with plenty of polymorphonuclear cells and mononuclear cells. (10×40)

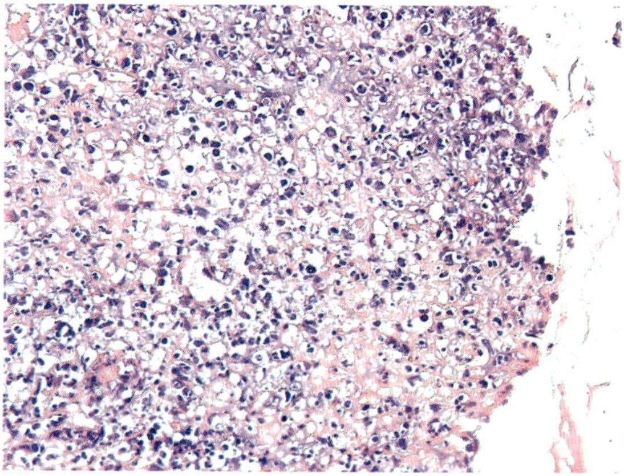

Fig.38 Fungal nasopharyngitis combind with atypical hyperplasia of nasopharyngeal mucosa (same case as in Fig.37 , another field)

Figure showed atypical hyperplasia of epithelial cells, cells arrangement disorder, like infiltration of certain malignant cells.(10×40)

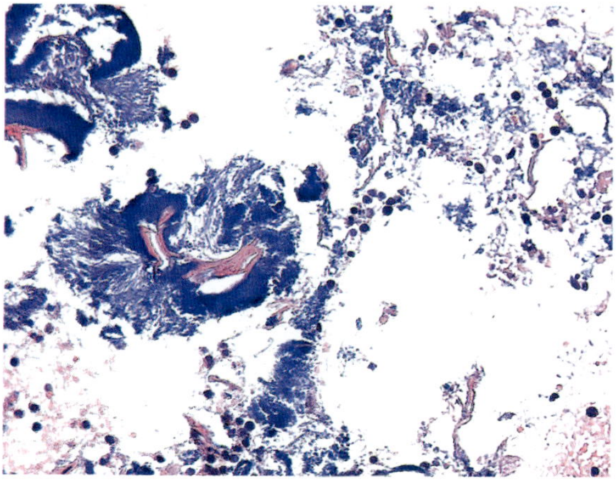

Fig.39 Necrotic inflammation of nasopharyux with plenty of fungus clusters in the purulent discharge

Male, 54 years old. Fugal clusters found in the flammatory exudate collected at the ulceration surface of chronic nasopharyngitis . (10×100)

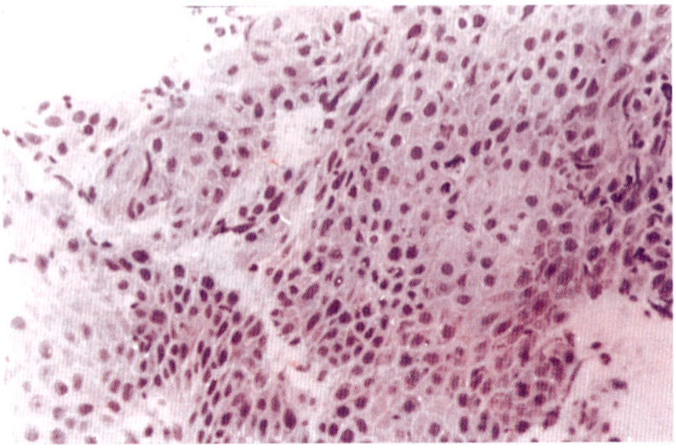

Fig.40 Overgrowth of squamous cell epithelium at nasopharynx (same patient as in Fig..39, another field)

Figure 40 showed that the ulcer border of nasopharyngeal mucosa was coverd by overgrowth of the squamous epithelium. (10×40)

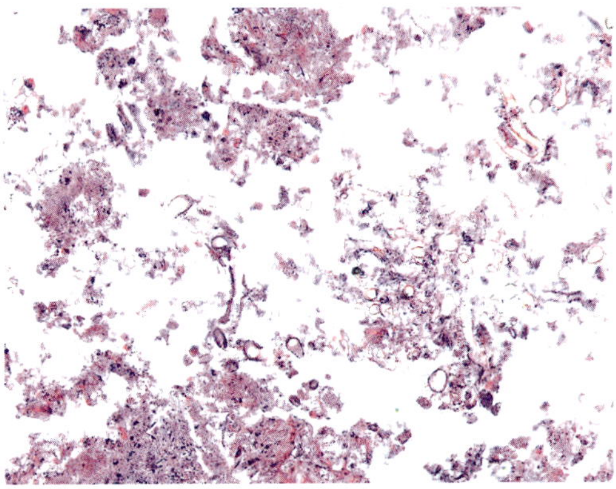

Fig.41 Moniliosis (Candidiasis) infection of nasopharynx

Female, 46 years old. Follow-up checking about one year after radiotherapy revealed a mild proliferation of granulation tissue over the left posterior wall of nasopharynx.

Figure 41 showed both fungal hyphae and spores seen in the inflammatory exudate. Oil immersion microscopy showed a narrow linkage present between the hyphae which is coincident to the diagnostic criteria of a candida hypha. In addition, nutritional vesiculae were obtained in longitudinal sections and granules or vesicle-like sunstance were seen in cross sections of the hyphae. Sporangiums and thick-capsule spores were seen in individual hypha. (10× 100)

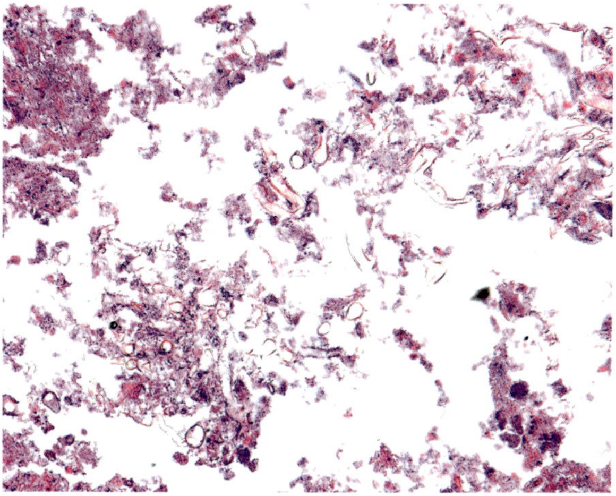

Fig.42 Moniliosis (Candidiasis) infection of nasopharynx (same case as in Fig.41, another field) (10×100)

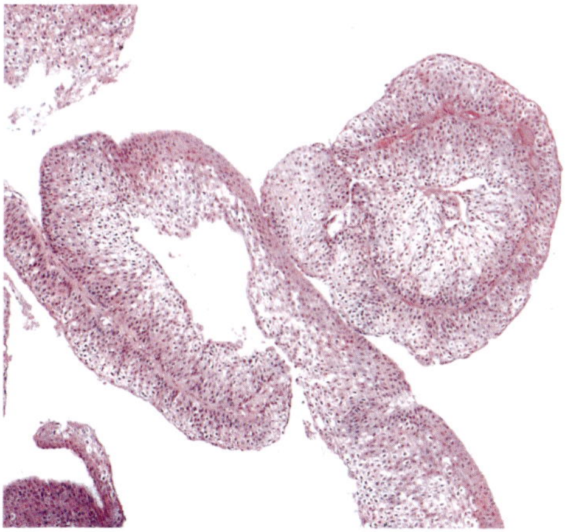

Fig.43 Squamous cell metaplasia and papillary proliferation of nasopharyngeal epithelium.

Male, 26 years old. A small nodule ($0.4 \times 0.4cm \times 0.6cm^3$) developed at the parietal wall of nasopharynx.

Figure 43 showed squamous cell metaplasia and papillary atypical hyperplasia of pseudostratified ciliated columnar epithelium.(10×10)

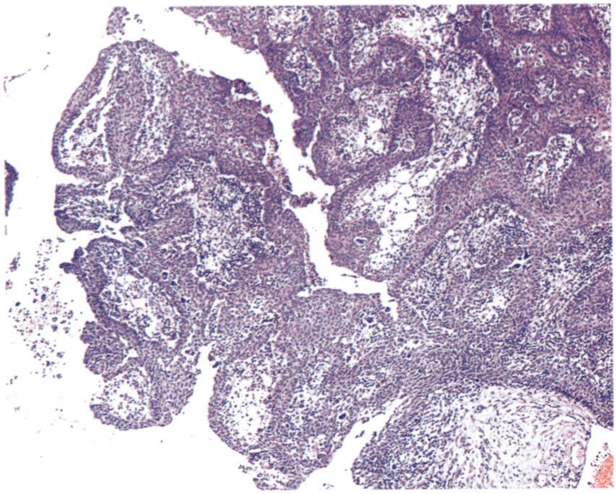

Fig.44 Papilloma of nasopharyngeal squamous cell epithelium

Male, 50 years old. A tumor growth was found at the right side parietal wall of nasopharynx during a mass survey, The surface of tumor mass was rough and granular.

Figure 44 showed papillary hyperplasia of squamous epithelium. A few capillaries and connective tissue were seen as the axis at the central part of the papilla.

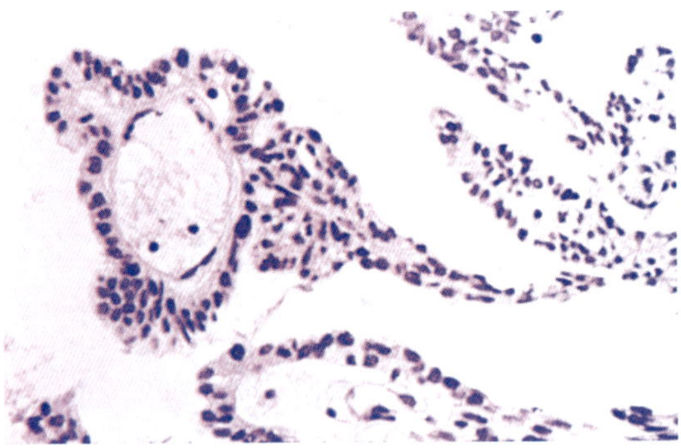

Fig.45 Papillary adenoma at nasopharyngeal fossa (similar to intraductal papilloma)

Male, 31 years old. Pharyngorhinoscopy showed: A node (0.2 cm×0.2 cm×0.1cm^3) with humid surface.

Figure shows: tumor cells, with papillary arrangement, having cores of fibrovascular stroma and presenting well-differentiated columnar and cuboidal epithelia, without inflitration. (10×40)

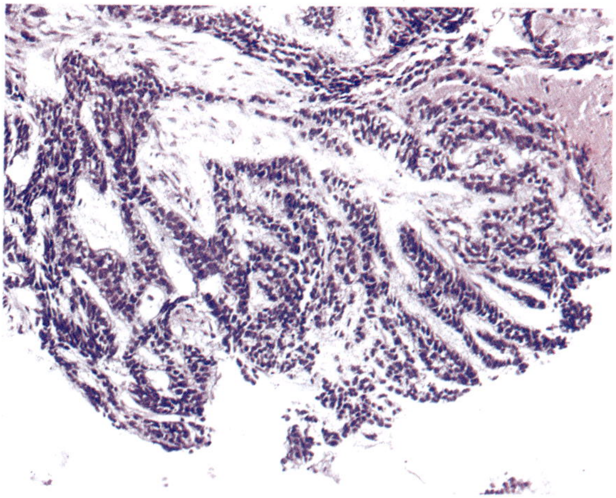

Fig.46 Adenoid basal cell carcinoma of nasopharynx (Adenoid basal cell epithelioma)

Male, 51 years old. Pharyngorhinoscopy shows an ulcer with rat-bite mark.He had a longer course of disease without metastasis of lymph nodes.

Figure shows: uniform tumor cells with adenoid arrangement, infiltrative growth and rare mitosis. (10×10)

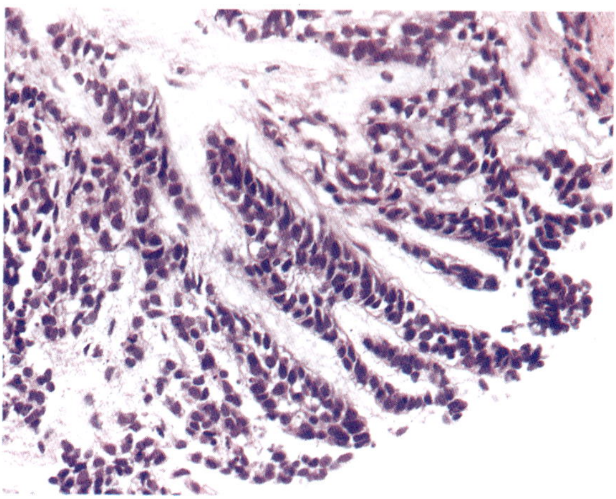

Fig.47 Adenoid basal cell carcinoma (adenoid basal cell epithelioma)of nasopharynx (same case as in Fig.46)

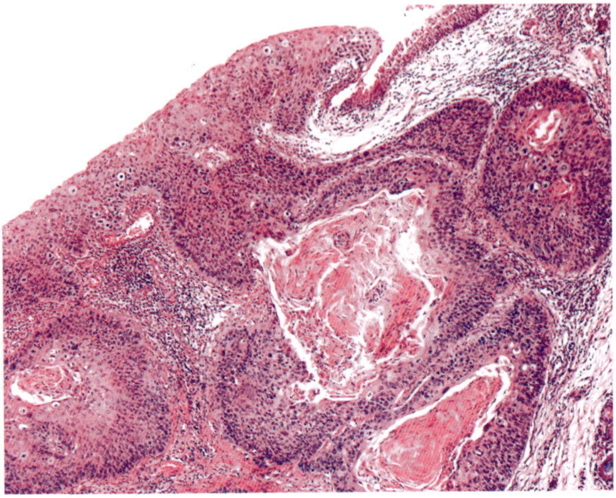

Fig.48 Squamous cell carcinoma grade I
(Keratinizing carcinoma) of nasopharynx

Male, 50 years old. Figure shows: the cancer cells show obvious keratinization, and there are complete keratinization of cancer-nests and keratinization of the cancer cells beyond 75%. (10×10)

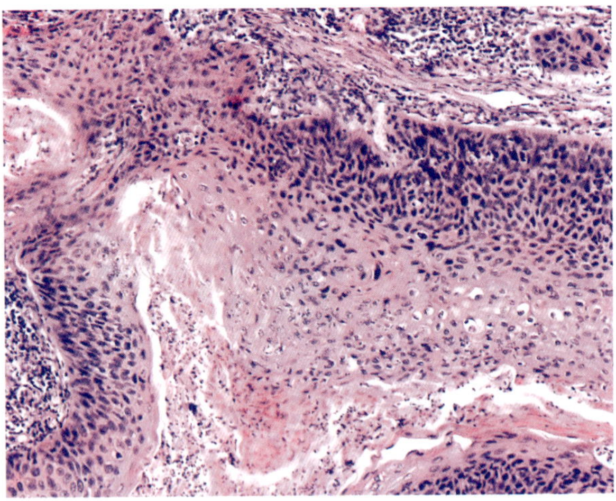

Fig.49 Squamous cell carcinoma grade I
(Keratinizing carcinoma) of nasopharynx(same case as in Fig.48)

Figure shows: well-differrntiated carcinomas can be seen the cancer cells have intercellular bridges and complete keratinization. (10×40)

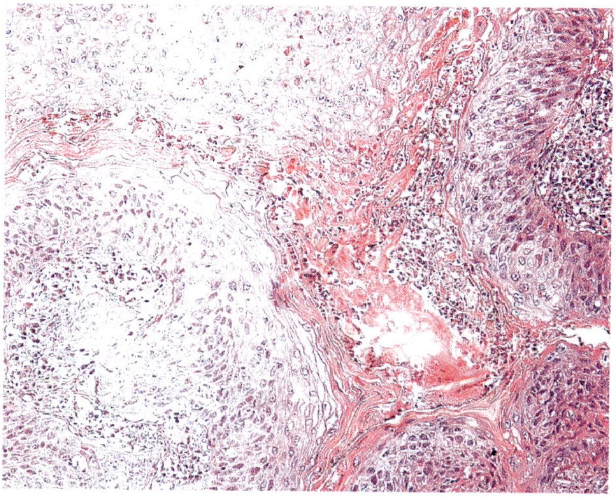

Fig.50 Squamous cell carcinoma grade I
(Keratinizing carcinoma) of nasopharynx(same case as in Fig.48)

Figure shows: the cancer-nests are surrounded by esosinophilic karetoprotein. (10×10)

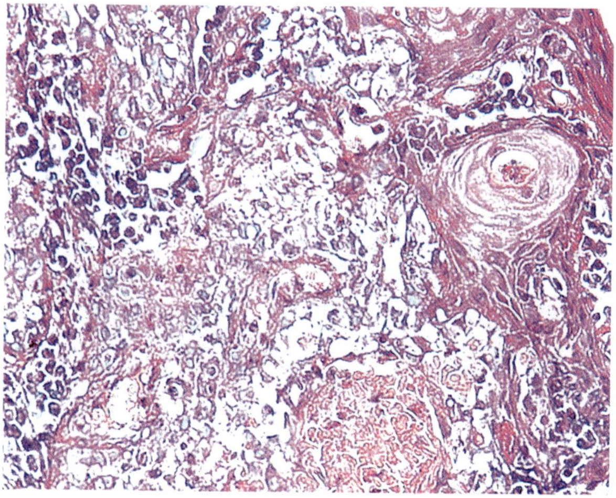

Fig.51 Squamous cell carcinoma grade I
(Keratinizing carcinoma) of nasopharynx (same case as in Fig.50)

Figure shows well-differentiated cancer cells forming keratin pearl. (10×40)

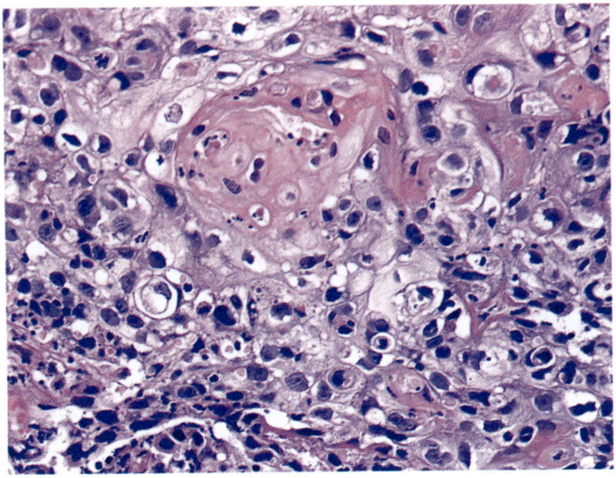

Fig.52 Squamous cell carcinoma grade II (Keratinizing carcinoma) of nasopharynx

Male, 48 years old. Figure shows: squamous cell dysplasia in one place, and arranged in nests and cords with breakthrough of the basement membrane(invasive growth). Polygonal and well-differentiated cancer cells with abundant cytoplasm and intercellular bridges, and keratinizing cells are nearly 50%. (10×40)

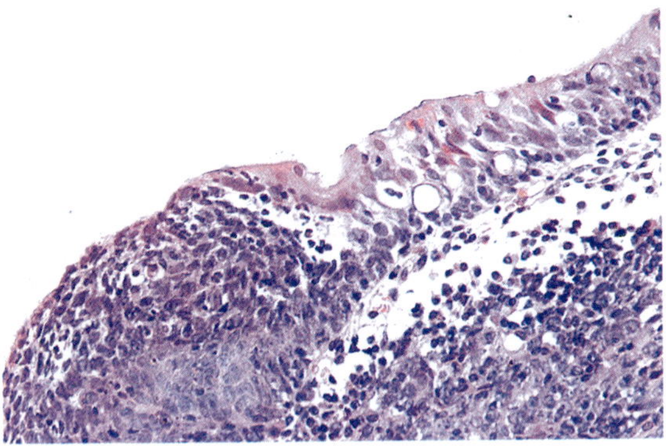

Fig.53 Atypical hyperplasia of columnar cells with malignant transformation in nasopharynx (carcinoma in situ)

Female, 44 years old. Figure shows: the layers of pseudostratified ciliated columnar epithelia increasing, basal cells with active hyperplasia infiltrating the whole layers of epithelia and becoming carcinoma in situ with several tens of layers and disorderly arrangement. (10×40)

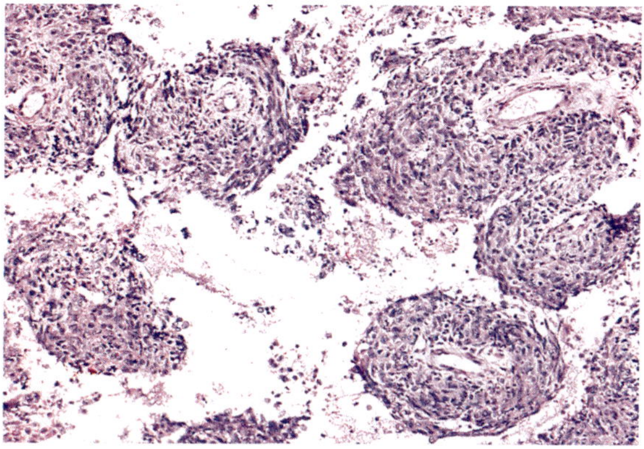

Fig.54 Squamous cell carcinoma grade III of nasopharynx (Non–keratinizing carcinoma)

Female, 67 years old. Figure shows: tumor cells with papillary growth, the papillary centers are composed of cores of fibrovascular stroma in the transverse section. Gross Figure is cauliflowers type of NPC. (10×10)

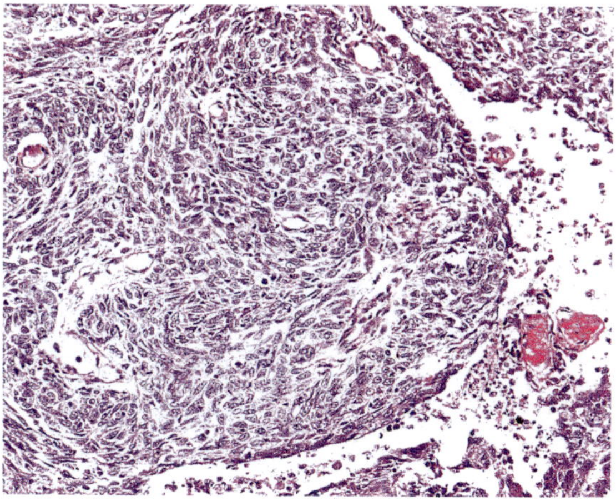

Fig.55 Squamous cell carcinoma grade III (same case as in Fig.54)

Figure shows: the cancer cells are arranged in papilloses and nests. Polygonal, spindle and oval cancer cells with clear border, rough chromosomes and no keratinizing, the scales of nuclear-plasma enlarge, the mitoses can be seen occasionally. (10×40)

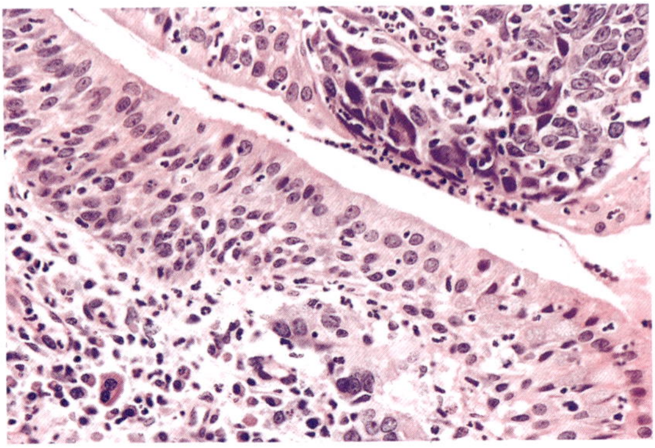

Fig.56 Atypical hyperplasia of columnar cells at nasopharyngeal fossa with malignant transformation to poorly-differentiated carcinoma

Female, 47 years old. Figure shows: the columnar epithelia dysplasia of unilateral glandular tube, with the larger scale of nuclear-plasma, varying size, hyperchromatic, and disorderly arrangement. The columnar epithelia invade to lamina propia, and become invasive carcinoma. (10×40)

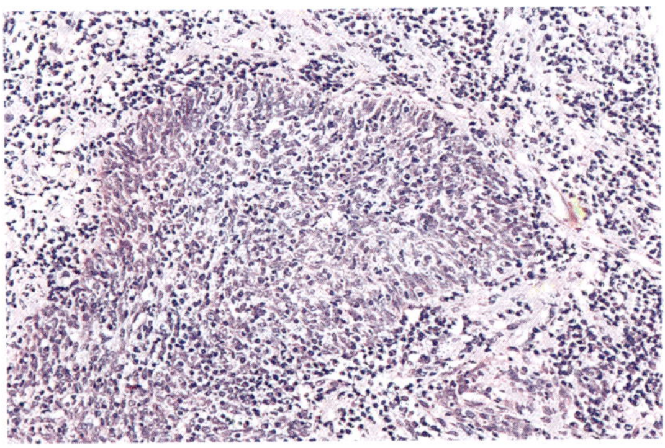

Fig.57 Squamous cell carcinoma grade III of nasopharynx (Non-keratinizing carcinoma)

Male, 49 years old. Figure shows: polygonal, round and oval cancer cells, with larger scale of nuclear-plasma, moderate cytoplasm, no karatinizing, are arranged in nest. Peripheral cells of the nests partly show palisading, similar as basal cells of squamous epithelia. The intercellular spaces of cancer nests inlay a few of lymphocytes; and the stroma is heavily infiltrated by lots of lymphocytes and plasmocytes. (10×10)

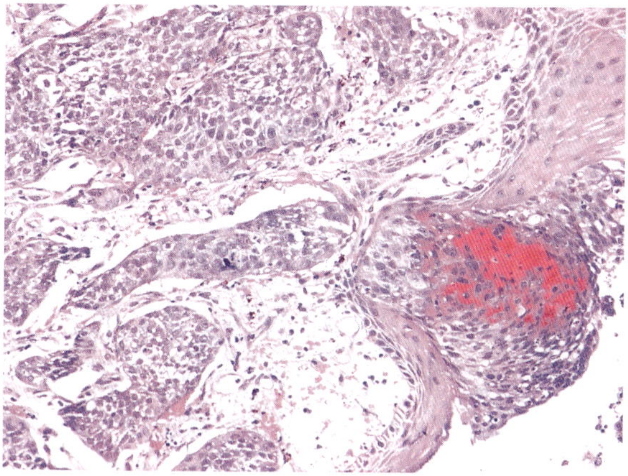

Fig.58 Squamous cell carcinoma grade III (Non-keratinizing carcinoma) of nasopharynx

Female, adult. Figure shows: the invasive cancer nests and cords invade under mucosal squamous epithelia, one of the cancer nests protruding from the surface, but bilateral epithelia are normal. Estimate the patient must be submucosa type of NPC. The surface of early cancer focus may be smooth. It is necessary to do a deeper biopsy in order to get the positive result easily. (10×10)

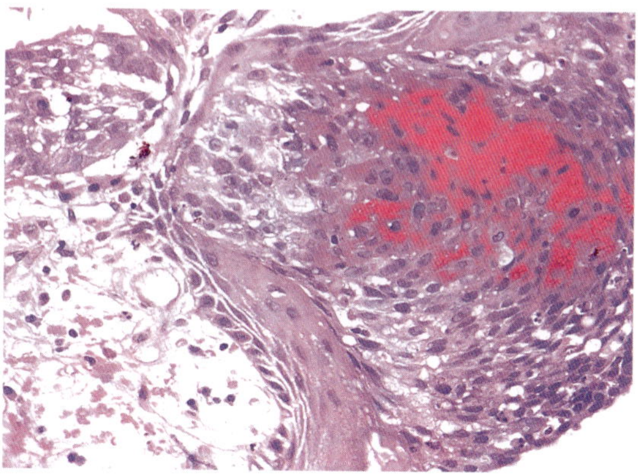

Fig.59 Squamous cell carcinoma, grade III of NPC (Non-keratinizing carcinoma)(same as Fig.58)

Figure shows: the image of cancer cords protruding from the surface under high power. (10×40)

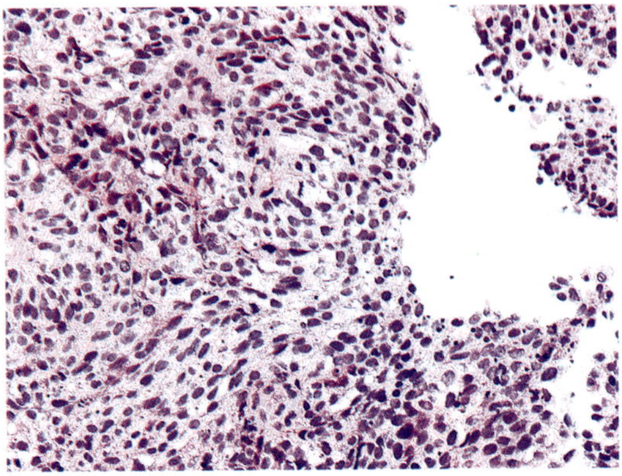

Fig.60 Squamous cell carcinoma grade III (Non-keratinizing carcinoma) of nasopharynx

Female, 49 years old. Figure shows: oval and round cancer cells (few polygonal), cancer pearls with concentric arrangement are surrounded by a few of spindle cancer cells. In the middle of the cancer pearl, there is a mitosis cancer cell (in metakinesis, chromosomes locating at the equatorial plane, and shaping as"—"). (10×40)

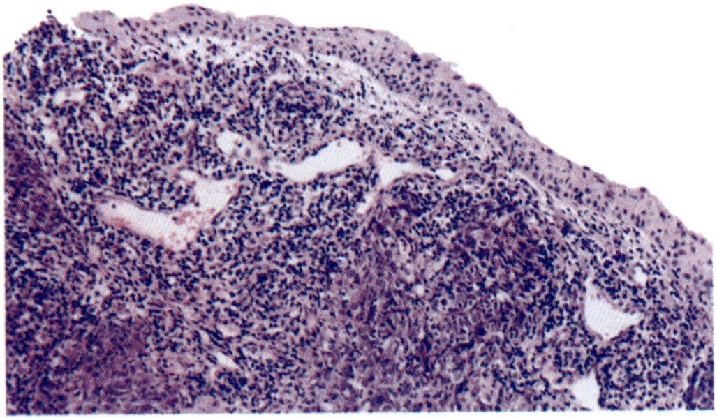

Fig.61 Pleomorphic carcinoma of nasopharynx, sub-mucosa type (Undifferentiated cell carcinoma)

Male, 24 years old. Figure shows: the invasive cancer nests and cords are under mucosal squamous epithelia, cancer cells are small and pleomorphic with scanty cytoplasm, indistinct cell border, part of vesicular nuclei. There is abundant stroma among cancer nests with reaction of lymphocytes, plasma cells and fibroblasts. (Lymphoepithetial carcinoma)(10×10)

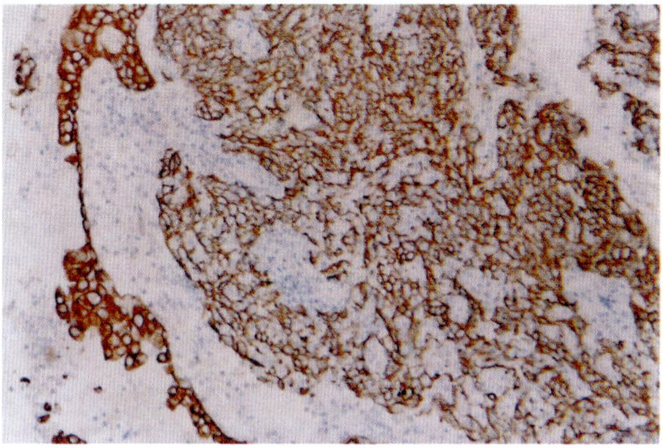

Fig.62 Pleomorphic cell carcinoma of nasopharynx, submucosa type

(undifferentiated cell and non-keratinizing carcinoma) (same case as in Fig.61)

Figure shows: Immunohistochemistry: CK(cytokeratin)(+) (10×20)

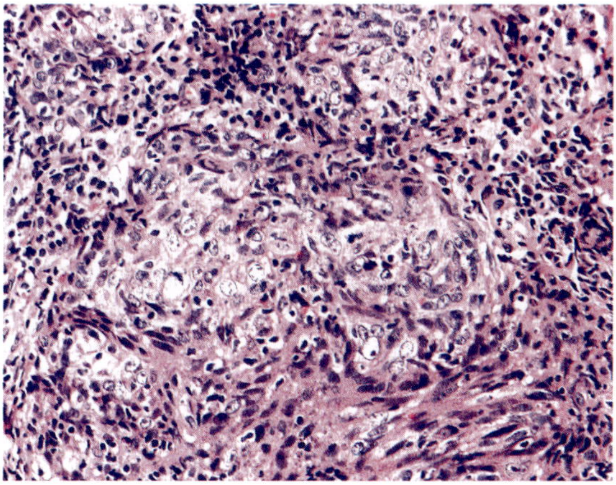

Fig.63 Pleomorphic cell carcinoma of nasopharynx (same case as in Fig.61 under high power)

Figure shows: the image of cancer nests magnified by high power lens. (10×40)

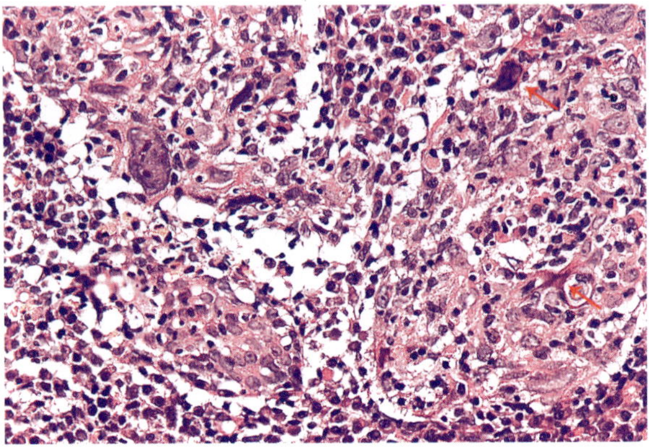

Fig.64 Pleomorphic cell carcinoma of nasopharynx
(same case as in Fig. 61, different field and under high power)

Figure shows: several mitoses indicate cancer cell active hyperplasia. (10×40)

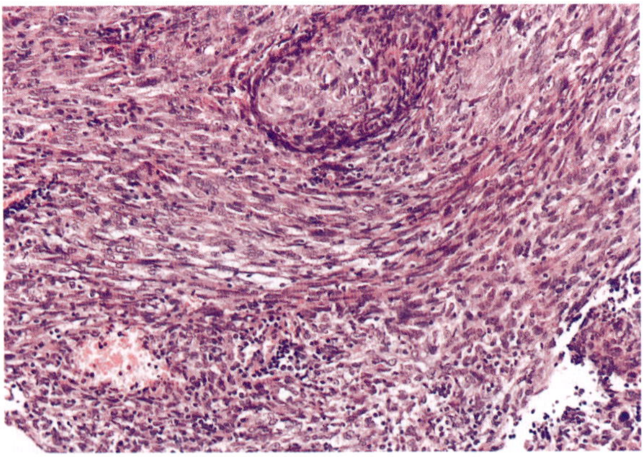

Fig.65 Spindle cell carcinoma of nasopharynx

Male, 72 years old. Figure shows: the cancer cells and nuclei are spindle, and have a feature of directional arrangement. Part of nuclei arrange in palisading, which are similar as fibrosarcoma and neurofibrosarcoma.However,there are no argentophilic fibers among cancer cells by argentophil fiber staining. The cancer cells surrounding the vascular stroma show palisading arrangement just as basal cells, and that suggests spindle cell carcinoma of nasopharynx and may be the subtype of poor-differentiated squmous cell carcinoma. (10×10)

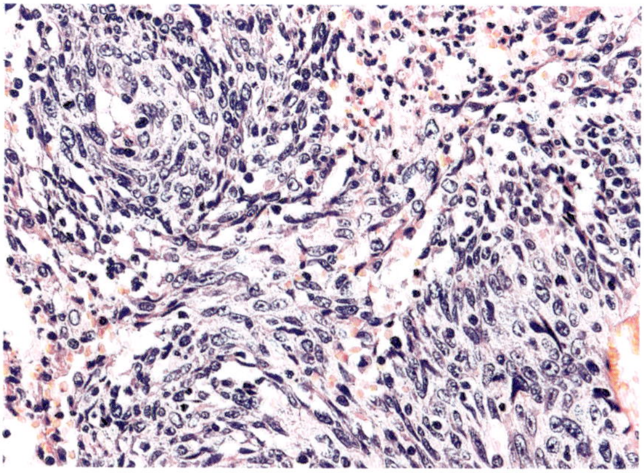

Fig.66 Spindle cell carcinoma of nasopharynx

Male, 43 years old. Figure shows: most cancer cells are splindle, with varying size, indistinct cell border and circinate or palisading arrangement. Basicranial bones are involved. He had NPC recurrence after radiotherapy 5 years. His condition had exacerbation rapidly, and then died. (10×40)

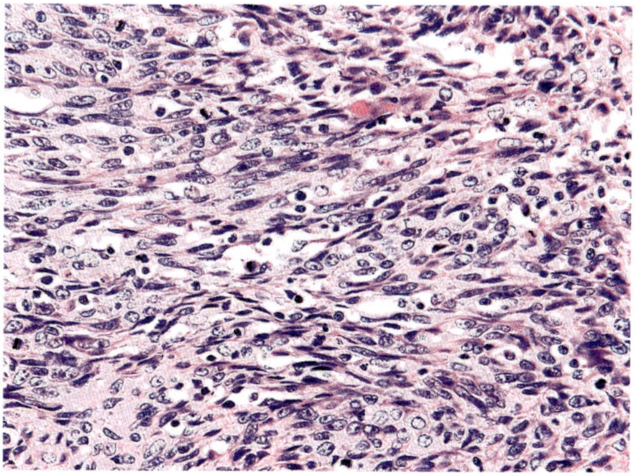

Fig.67 Spindle cell carcinoma of nasopharynx

Female, 32 years old. Figure shows: spindle cancer cells with interlacing arrangement are similar as fibrosarcoma. (10×40)

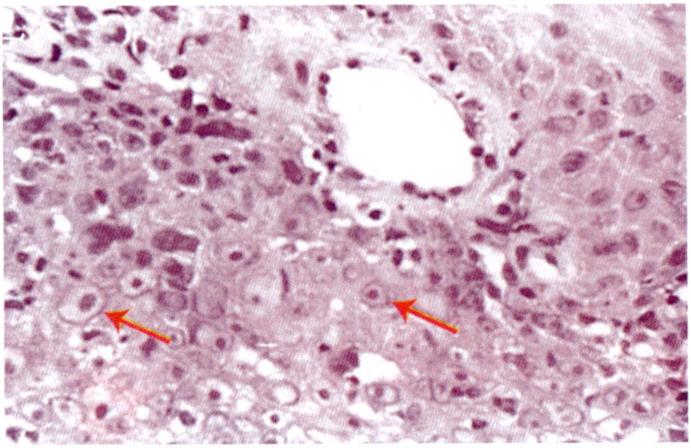

Fig.68 Basal cell hyperplasia of squamous epithelium and transformed to giant round cell carcinoma of nasopharynx

Male, 36 years old. Figure shows: the superficial squmous epithelia are orderly yet. The basement membrane has been destroyed in one place. The basal cells have active hyperplasia and infiltrate downwards. Giant round cancer cells, with the scale of nuclear-plasma enlarging, giant nucleoli, hypochromatic and vesicular nuclei, may originate from the basal cells of squamous epithelia. (10×40)

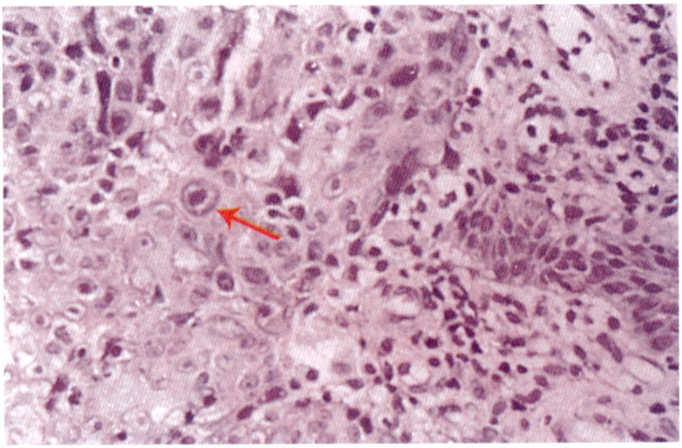

Fig.69 Basal cell hyperplasia of squamous epithelium and transformed to giant round cell carcinoma of nasopharynx (10×40)

Same case as in Fig.68, another field,the squamous epithelial basal cells on the right side are normal.

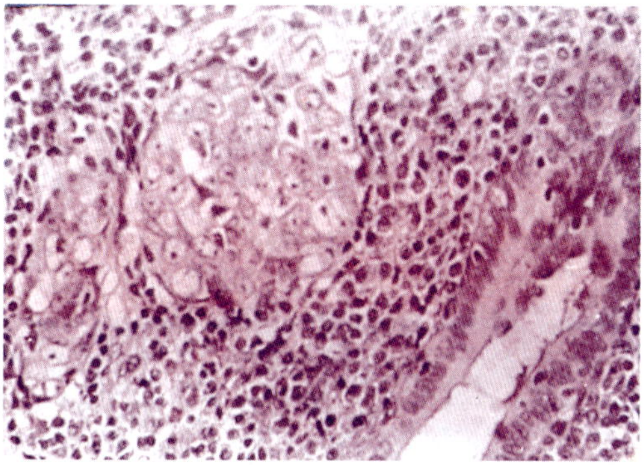

Fig.70 Atypical hyperplasia of glandular columnar cells and transformed into giant round cell carcinoma of nasopharynx (undifferentiated cell carcinoma of NPC)

Male, 36 years old. Figure shows: columnar epithelia of unilateral adenotubes hyperplasia arranging in multiple layers. The cells have prominent nucleoli and larger scale of nucleus-plasma. Another two solid adenotubes are instead by giant round cancer cells with vesicular nuclei. The border of cancer nests remains a few of spindle myoepithelia. Above-mention indicates that columnar epithelia atypical hyperplasia may transit to giant round cell carcinoma of nasopharynx. (10×40)

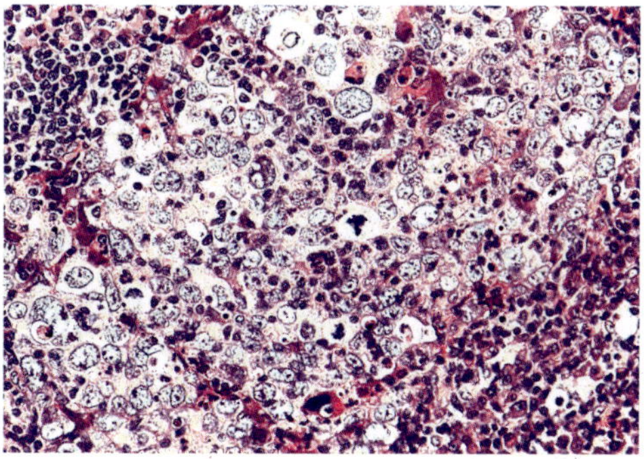

Fig.71 Giant round cell carcinoma of nasopharynx

Male, 67 years old. He had cervical lumps, the nasophayngeal neoplasm and nasal hemorrhage for one year more. Figure shows: the giant round cells have varying size, clear nuclei, prominent nucleoli, scanty cytoplasm and cluster arrangement. In the middle of the Figure, there is a cancer cell with a four-polar mitosis. (10×40)

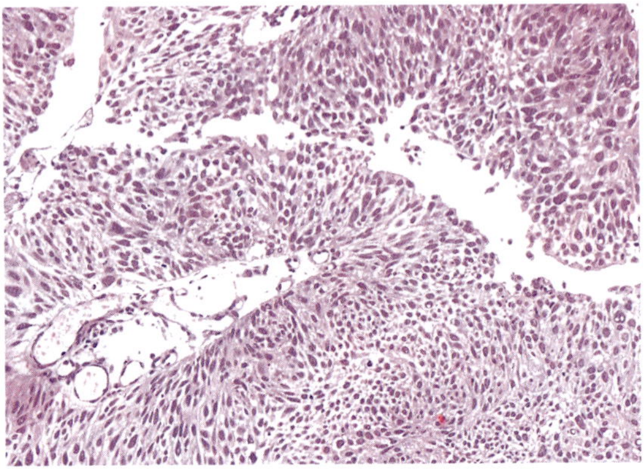

Fig.72 Squamous cell carcinoma (grade III) of nasopharynx (Non-keratinizing carcinoma)

Female, 48 years old. Figure shows: pseudostratified ciliated columnar epithelia of nasopharyngeal mucosal surface arise squmous metaplaisa, and then instead by countless layers of the cancer cells. The cancer cells arrange in atypical papillary shape with central cores of fibrovascular stroma. (10×10)

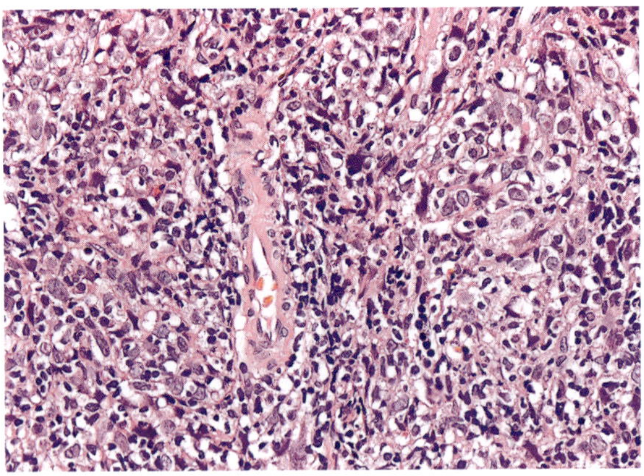

Fig.73 Squamous cell carcinoma (grade III) of nasopharynx (Non-keratinizing carcinoma) (same case as in Fig.72)

Figure shows: pleomorphic cancer cells with varying size, and cancer cells of giant nuclei.The case proves that some pleomorphic cancers exactly are poor-differentiated,anaplastic squamous carcinoma (10×40)

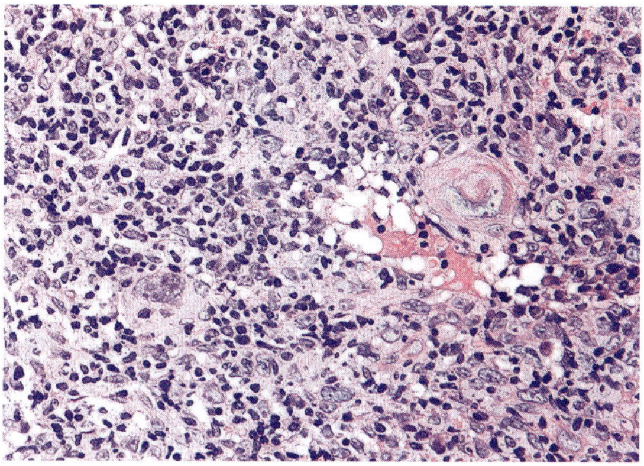

Fig.74 Pleomorphic cell carcinoma of nasopharynx (Non-keratinizing carcinoma)

Female, 72 years old. Figure shows: the carcinoma is composed of pleomorphic cancer cells. Round and polygonal cancer cells can be seen as well as giant or polynuclear cancer cells. The cancer cells arrange diffusely. Two giant cancer cells with vesicular nucleoli and cytophagous phenomenon can be seen. (10×40)

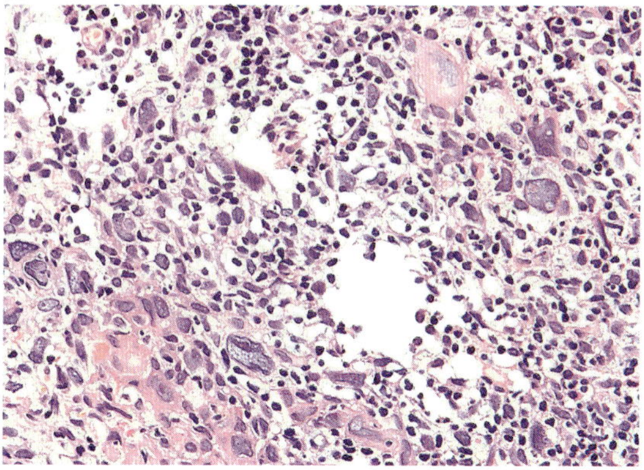

Fig.75 Pleomorphic cell carcinoma of nasopharynx (Non-keratinizing carcinoma)

Male, 65 years old. He had tinnitus, hypoacusis, with lumps of bilateral necks. Necrotic neoplasm could be seen by pharyngorhinoscopy. Figure shows: obviously pleomorphic cancer cells with varying size; and there are a lot of giant cancer cells. (10×40)

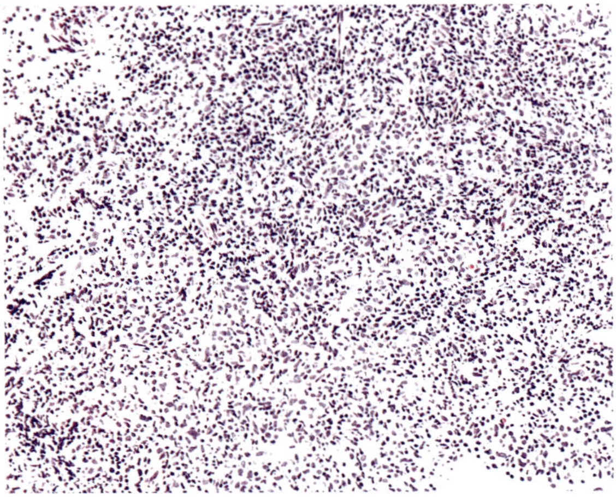

Fig.76 Undifferentiated cell carcinoma of nasopharynx

Male, 36 years old. Figure shows: small and round cancer cells have cord arrangement. (10×10)

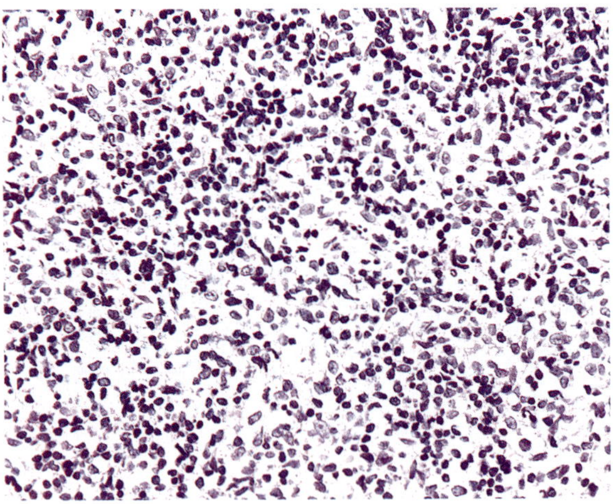

Fig.77 Undifferentiated cell carcinoma of nasopharynx

Male, 60 years old. Figure shows: cancer cells are small, round, polygonal and kemeloid with scanty cytoplasm, with hyperchromatic nuclei and diffuse arrangement, epithelial origin can't be identified. (10×40)

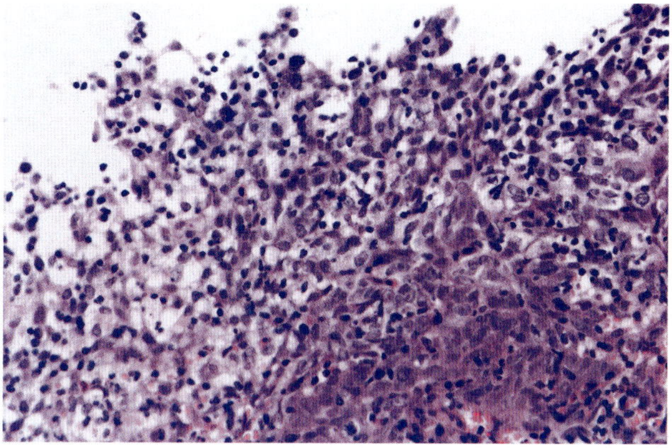

Fig.78 After radiotherapy recurrence of Squamous cell carcinoma (grade III)

Male, 41 years old. The case is the patient with recurrence of NPC after radiotherapy. Figure shows: the cancer cells grow actively, with arrangement of multiple layers (10×40)

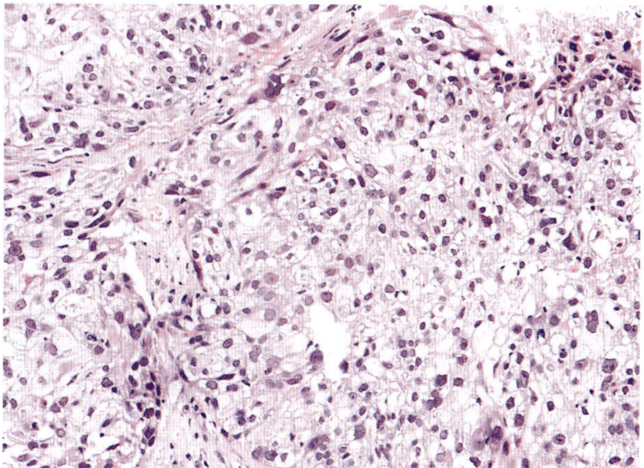

Fig.79 Clear cell carcinoma of nasopharynx

Male, 32 years old. Figure shows: the cancer cells arrange in nests, with hyperchromatic nuclei of varying size, and clear cytoplasm just as vacuoles. (10×10)

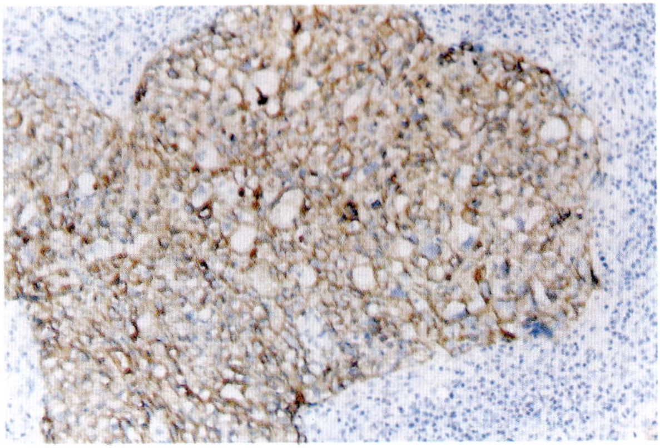

Fig.80 Clear cell carcinoma of Nasopharynx.
(same case as in Fig.79)
Immunohistochemistry: CK(Cytokeratin) (+) (10×20)

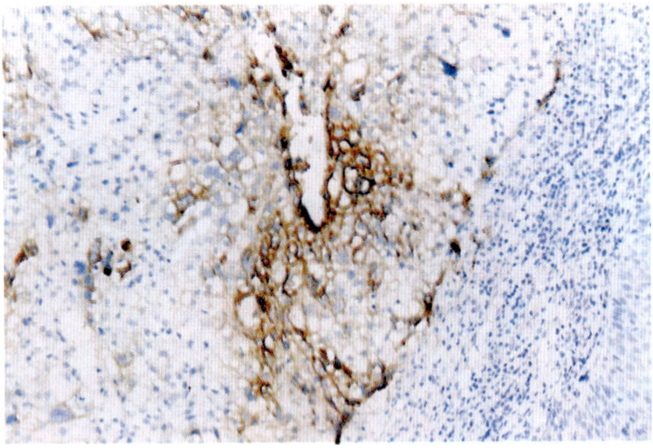

Fig.81 Clear cell carcinoma of nasopharynx.
(same case as in Fig. 80)
Immunohistochemistry:CEA(+)(Carcinoembryonic antigen) (10×20)

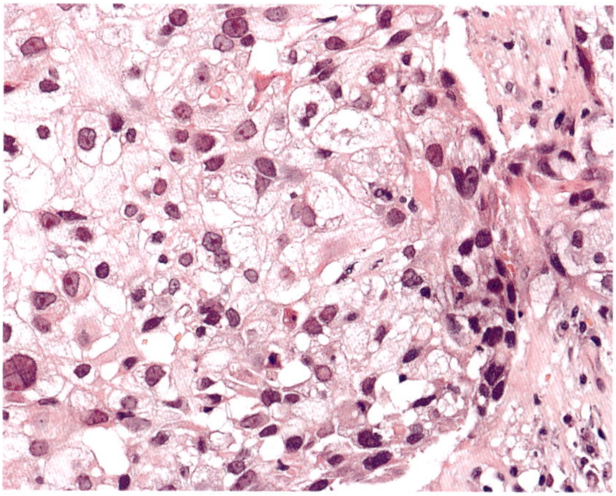

Fig.82 Clear cell carcinoma of nasopharynx
(same case as in Fig.79, under high power)

Figure shows: cancer cells with especially abundant cytoplasm as clear as vesicular. The contour of vesicular cytoplasm is left because of glycogen dissolution in the process of making slides.This type was confirmed to be a subtype of squamous carcinoma. (10×40)

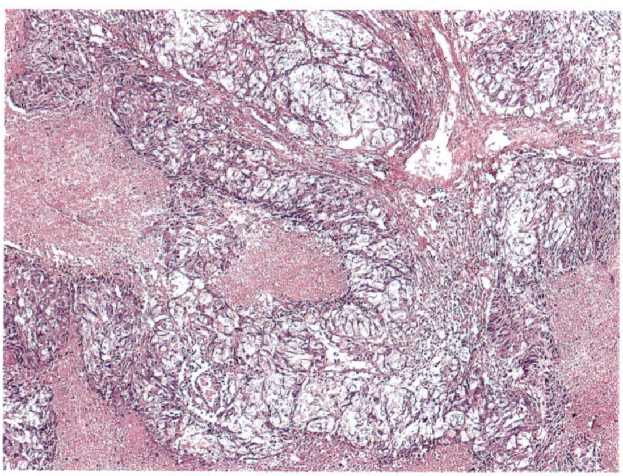

Fig.83 Poorly-differentiated carcinoma of nasopharynx
(adenoid type)

Male, 53 years old. Figure shows: the cancer cells arrange as glandular tubes. There are some pale red stained materials of liquefaction necrosis in tubal cavities. (10×10)

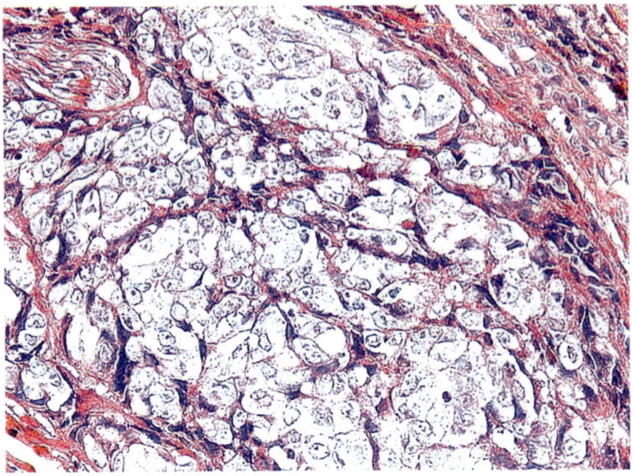

Fig.84 Poorly-differentiated carcinoma of nasopharynx (adenoid type) (same case as in Fig.83, under high power)

Figure shows: there are two types of the cancer cells: the cells of one type are giant round cancer cells with clear nuclei and cytoplasm; the cells of the other type are spindle cancer cells with hyperchromatic nuclei, and the body inlay each other. The cells arrange in irregular glandular tubes under low power. (10×40)

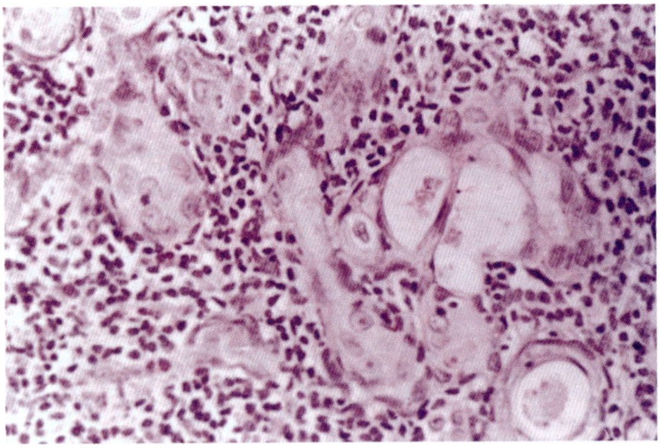

Fig.85 Adenosquamous carcinoma of nasopharynx

Male, 50 years old. He had tinnitus of the right ear, slight nasal hemorrhage, and the nodular masses of the right parietal nasopharynx and the right neck. Figure shows: cancer cells arrange as irregular glandular tubes, and part of them tend to keratinizing. There are keratinizing materials piling in glandular cavities. (10×40)

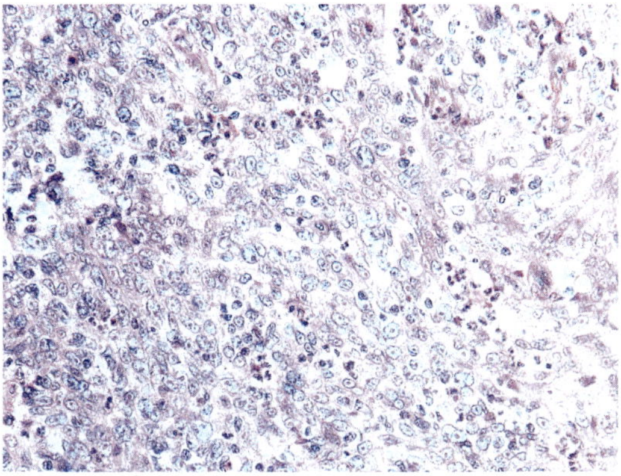

Fig.86 Pleomorphic cell carcinoma of nasopharynx

Female, 40 years old. Figure shows: big and round cancer cells with prominent nucleoli, clear nuclei and diffuse arrangement, mix with small and round cells, polygonal cells and hyperchromatic cells with giant nuclei. There are no fibers surrounding cancer nests. (10×20)

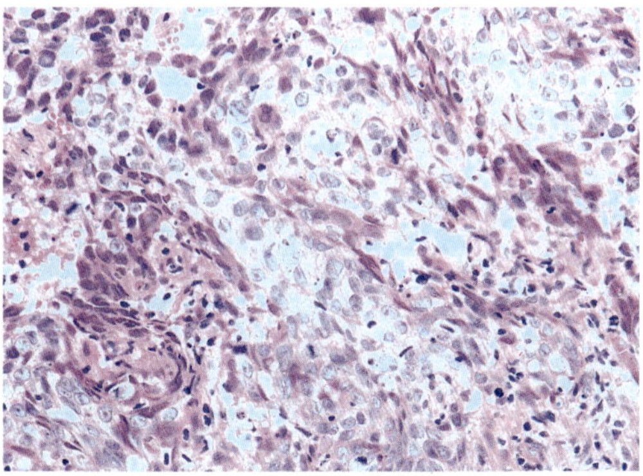

Fig.87 Poorly-differentiated carcinoma of nasopharynx (Mixed-cell type)

Male, 45 years old. He had tinnitus, headache, nasal obstruction,and nasal hemorrhage for one month more,and ulcerous neoplasm of parietal wall of nasophaynx could be seen by pharyngorhinoscopy. Figure shows: there are two types of the cells,one of them are cancer cells with hypochromatic nuclei,clear and abundant cytoplasm, distinct cell border and arranging in irregular adenoid nests;the other type are spindle cancer cells with hyperchromatic nuclei, eosinophilic cytoplasm and directional arrangement. The cells distribute into hypochromatic cancer nests. (10×40)

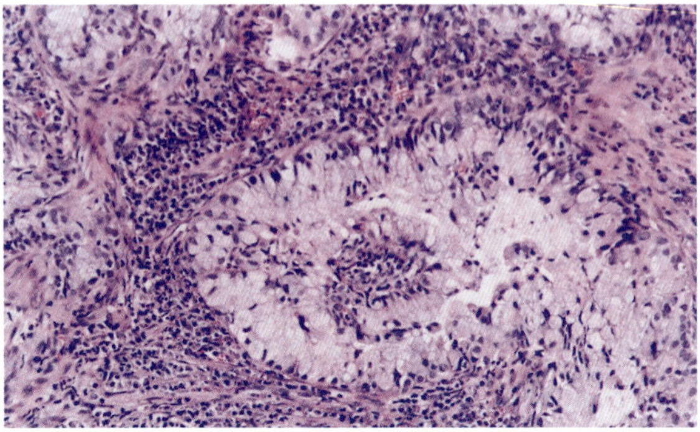

Fig.88 Adenocarcinoma of nasopharynx (columnar cell carcinoma of nasopharnx)

Male, 60 years old. Figure shows: there are high columnar cancer cells with oval nuclei and irregular glandular arrangement.Moderate lymphocytes and plasma cells infiltrate in the stroma. (10×40)

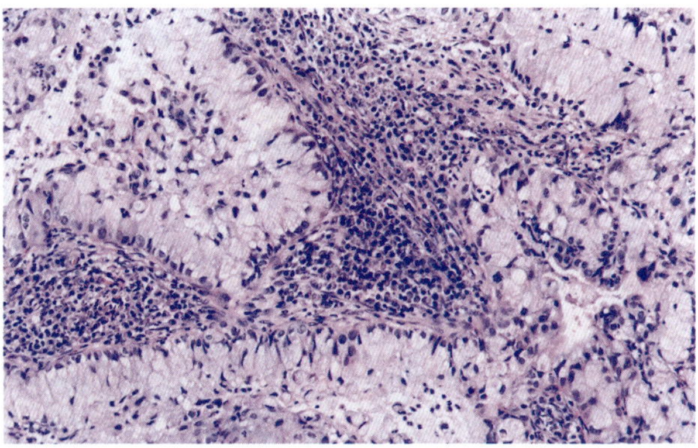

Fig.89 Adenocarcinoma of nasopharynx

Female,68 years old.She had left headache for four months more,nasal hemorrhage and deaf ears for two weeks.The invasive neoplasm of parietal nasophaynx could be seen by pharyngorhinoscopy.

Figure shows: columnar, high cuboidal or round cancer cells with varying size of hypochromatic nuclei, prominent nucleoli and chromatinic granules, arrange in glandular cavities. (10×40)

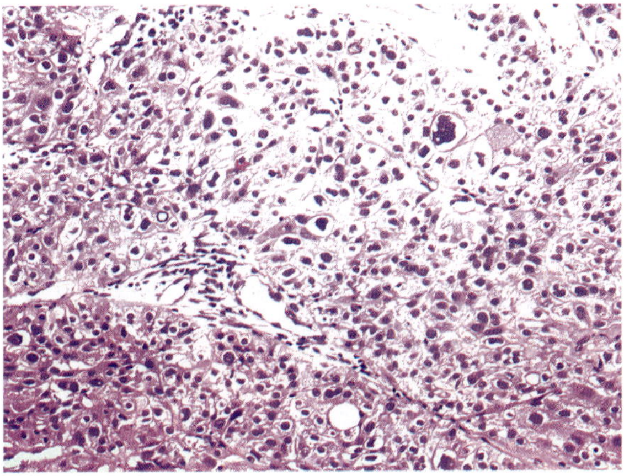

Fig.90 Adenocarcinoma of nasopharynx
(same case as in Fig.89, anothe field)

Figure shows: the cancer cells arrange in the solid cords, with obviously atypical and highly hyperchromatic nuclei, there are secretory vacuoles in cytoplasm.(10×20)

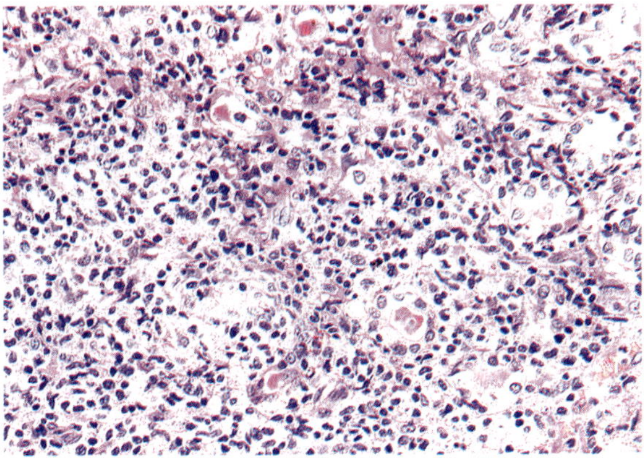

Fig.91 Small acinar adenocarcinoma of nasopharynx

Female, 22 years old. Figure shows: cuboidal and round cancer cells with visible nucleoli partly arrange in well-differentiated acinae,back-to-back patterns are common and the cancer cells diffusedly infiltrate among acinae. (10×20)

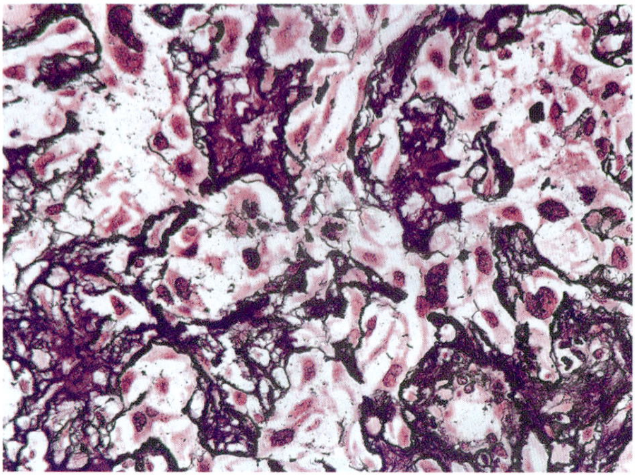

Fig.92 Small acinar adenocarcinoma of nasopharynx (same case as in Fig.91)

Figure shows: there are argentophilic fibers incompletely surrounding acinae by argentophilic fibers staining. (10×40)

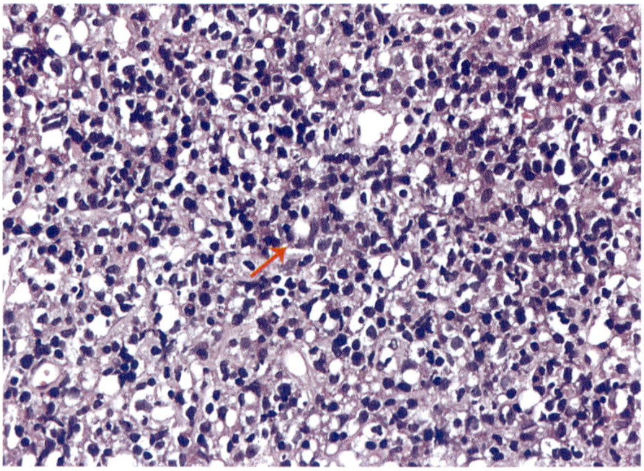

Fig.93 Poorly-differentiated small acinar adenocarcinoma of nasopharynx

Male, 57 years old. Figure shows: The small cancer cells diffusedly distribute under low power lens. The case can be misdiagnosed as lymphoma easily and can be distinguished from it by argentophilic fibers staining and careful observation through high power lens. (10×10)

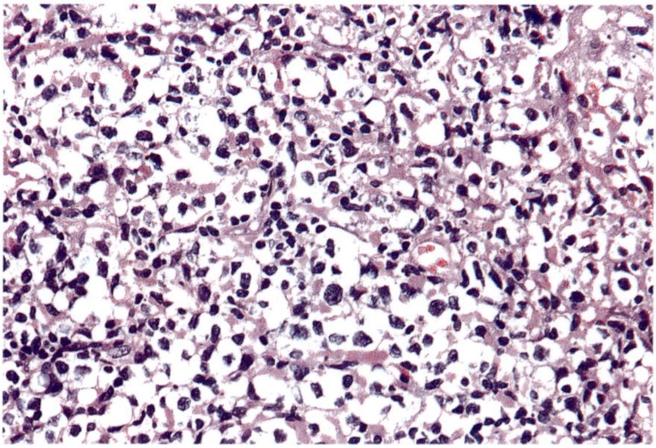

Fig.94 Poorly-differentiated small acinar adenocarcinoma of nasopharynx (same case as in Fig.93)

Figure shows: irregularly round cancer cells with varying size, hyperchromatic nuclei, vacant and clear cytoplasm or secretory vacuoles. Part nuclei are asymmetry, and a few of them become signet-ring cancer cells. However, there are no typical glandular structures. (10×40)

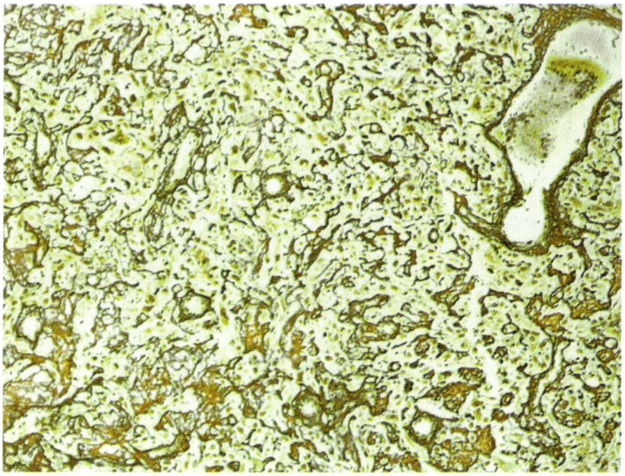

Fig.95 Poorly-differentiated small acinar adenocarcinoma of nasopharynx (same case as in Fig.93,argentophilic fibers staining.)

Figure shows: the cancer cells can be comparted into irregular solid acinae or cords by brown-black argentophilic fibers. The case may be distinguished from lymphoma by this image. (10×10)

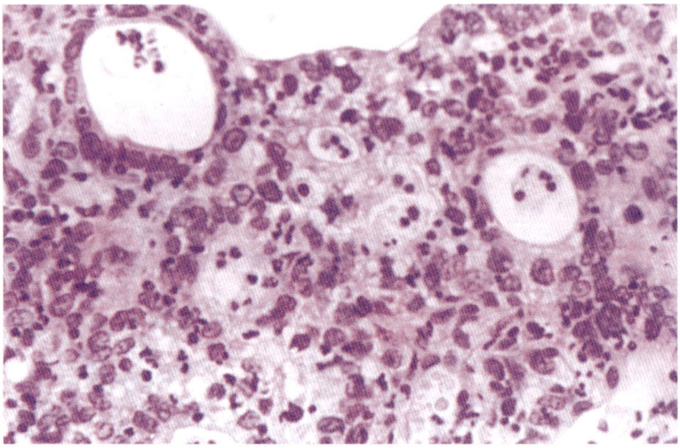

Fig.96 Small acinar adenocarcinoma of nasopharynx

Female, 37 years old. She had nasal hemorrage and jugular lumps. The nodular neoplasm could be seen by pharyngorhinoscopy. Figure shows: cuboidal cancer cells with irregularly acinar arrangement, back-to-back patterns can be seen among acinae. The cancer cells appear invasive growth. (10×40)

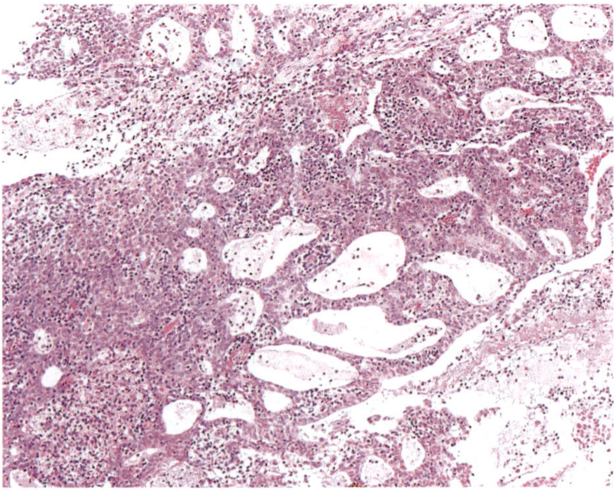

Fig.97 Small acinar adenocarcinoma of nasopharynx

Female, adult. Figure shows: cuboidal cancer cells arrange in dilatational acinae. Back-to-back patterns can be seen. Rosy and amorphous secretory materials accumulate in acinar cavities. (10×10)

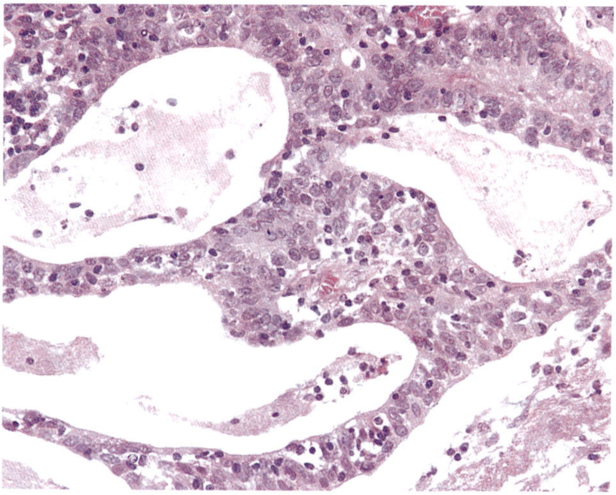

Fig.98 Small acinar adenocarcinoma of nasopharynx (same case as in Fig.97, under high power) (10×40)

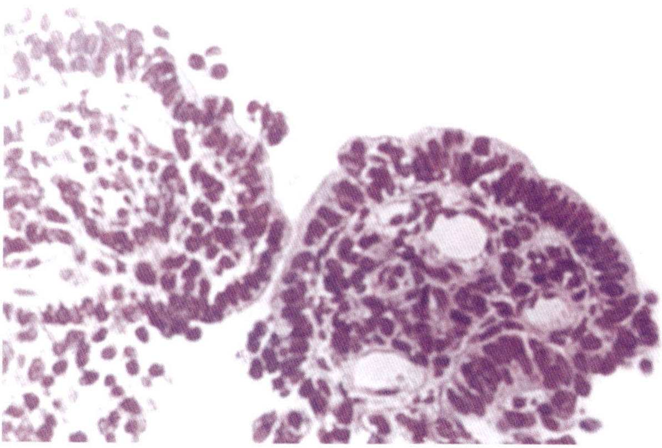

Fig.99 Papillary adenocarcinoma of nasopharynx

Male, 45 years old. He had lumps of the right neck. Cauliflower type of the neoplasm of right parietal wall of nasophaynx could be seen by pharyngorhinoscopy. Figure shows: cancer cells are with papillary arrangement. Scattered cancer cells invade the papillary cores of fibrovascular stroma(10×40)

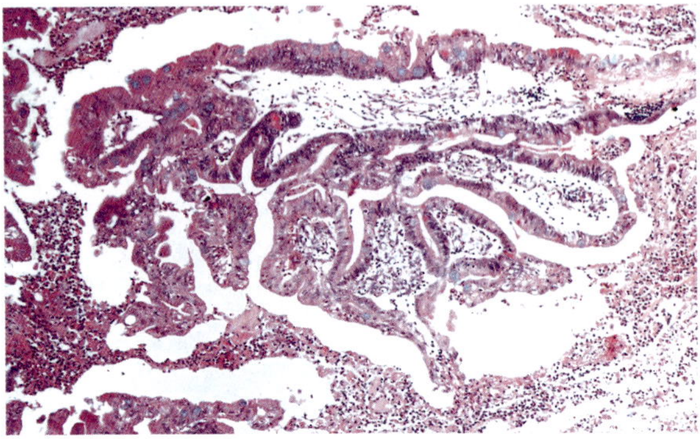

Fig.100 Papillary adenocarcinoma of nasopharynx

Male, 50 years old. He had nasal hemorrhage in April 1979.The neoplasm ($0.5\times0.5\times0.3cm^3$) could be seen by pharyngorhinoscopy. But the biopsy was negative. Seven months later, he suddenly had nasal hemorrhage, the pathological biopsy was: papillary adenocarcinoma of nasopharynx. The effect of radiotherapy of the whole procedure was not good.

Figure shows: the cancer cells have irregularly papillary glandular arrangement and invasive growth. Columnar cancer cells can be seen with varying size, atypical and hyperchromatic nuclei, and prominent nucleoli. Pathological mitoses can be seen occasionally. (10×10)

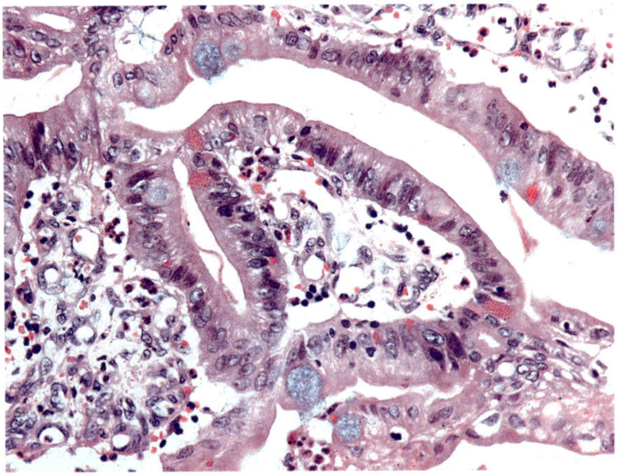

Fig.101 Papillary adenocarcinoma of nasopharynx (same case as in Fig.100, another field) (10×40)

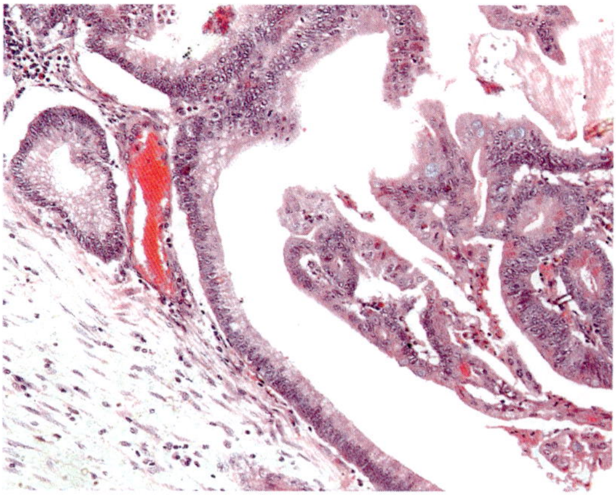

Fig.102 Papillary adenocarcinoma of nasopharynx (same case as in Fig.100) (10×40)

The magnified image of papillary parts by high power lens.

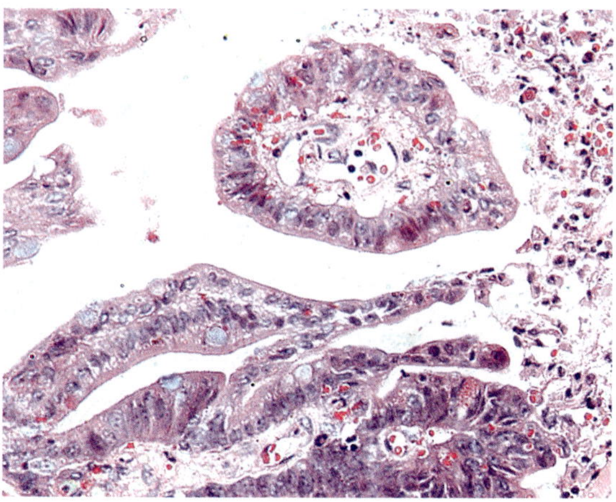

Fig.103 Papillary adenocarcinoma of nasopharynx (same case as in Fig.102,another field)

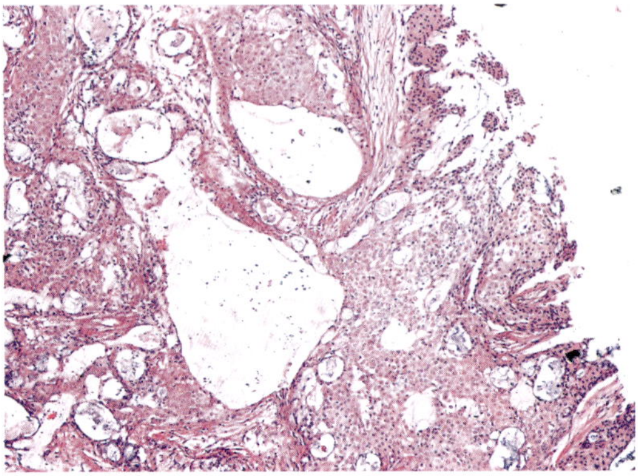

Fig.104　Mucoepidermoid carcinoma of nasopharynx

Male, 63 years old. He had nasal obstruction, mucous nasal secretion and nasopharyngeal lumps for three years, and no jugular metastasis. Figure shows: part of the cancer cells are similar as squamous epithelia; and part of them with azury mucous secretion and asymmetry nuclei.The cancer cells arrange are adenoid in nests and infiltrating growth. (10×10)

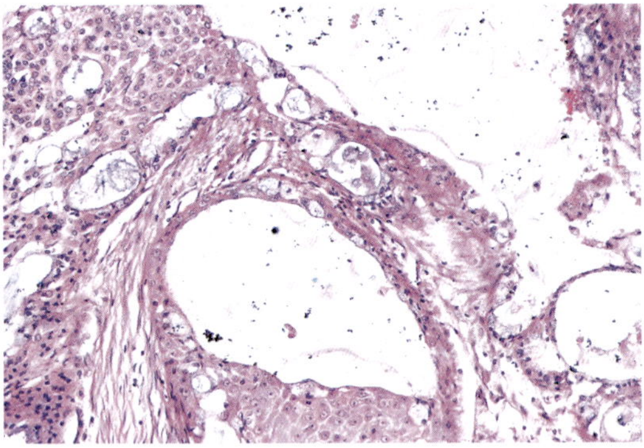

Fig.105　Mucoepidermoid carcinoma of nasopharynx (same case as in Fig.104, under high power)

Figure shows: round cancer cells have clear, abundant and azury cytoplasm. Some nuclei are asymmetry and hyperchromatic, as well as irregular shapes. Those are adenocarcinoma cells; parts of them are squamous cancer cells. (10×40)

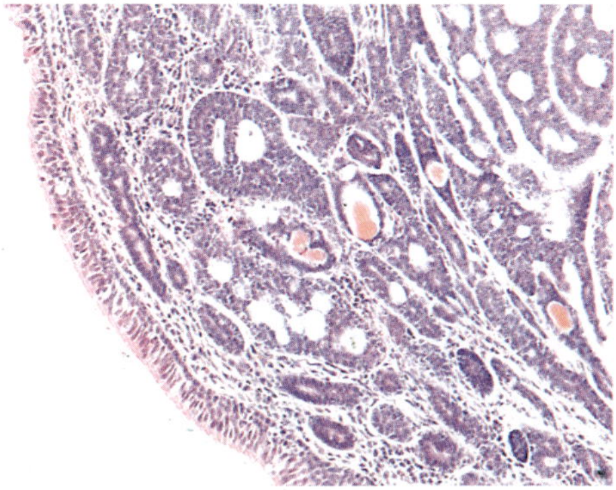

Fig.106 Adenoid cystic carcinoma of nasopharynx (cylindroma)

Male, 30 years old. He had nasal obstruction and nasal hemorrhage for four years more. The nodular neoplasm ($2 \times 3 \times 3cm^3$) of parietal nasopharynx could be seen by pharyngorhinoscopy.

Figure shows: pseudostratified ciliated columnar epithelia of nasopharyngeal mucosal surface are intact, glandular groups in cribriform structure infiltrate under epithelia; ethmoidal foramen contain mucohyaline materials. The small and round lymphocytes infiltrate stroma. (10×10)

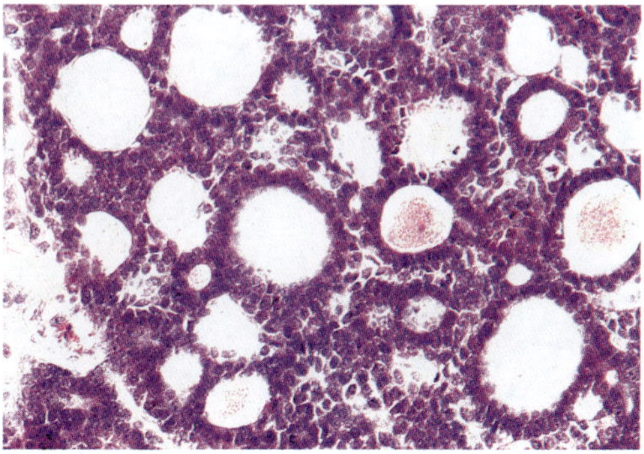

Fig.107 Adenoid cystic carcinoma of nasopharynx (same case as in Fig.106, under high power)

Figure shows: the tumor has two types of glands: (1) tubules containing red secretory materials; (2) tubules containing azury secretory materials.(10×40)

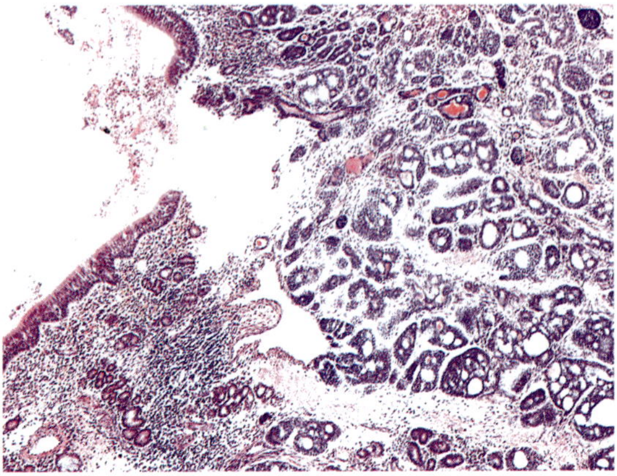

Fig.108 Adenoid cystic carcinoma of nasopharynx (cylindroma)

Male, 48 years old. Figure shows: the epithelia of mucosal surface have ulcerous hemorrhage in one place. The others are similar as Fig.106. (10×10)

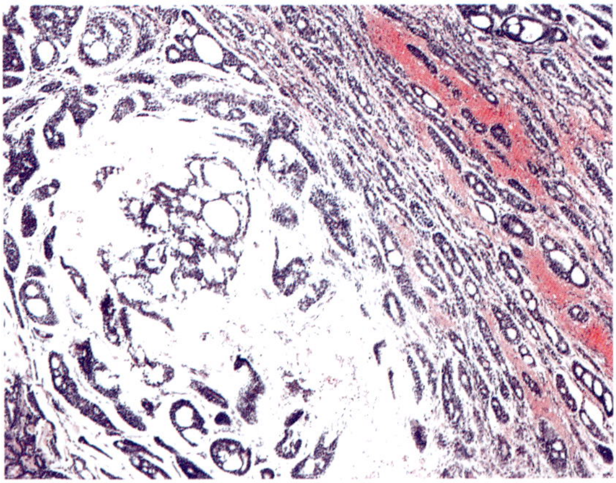

Fig.109 Adenoid cystic carcinoma of nasopharynx (same case as in Fig.108, another field)

Figure shows: the cancer cells arrange in solid cords, and stromal fibers are hyperplasia. As biopsy if the taken tissue is too little and without cribriform structure, the morphosis is similar to simple carcinoma. (10×10)

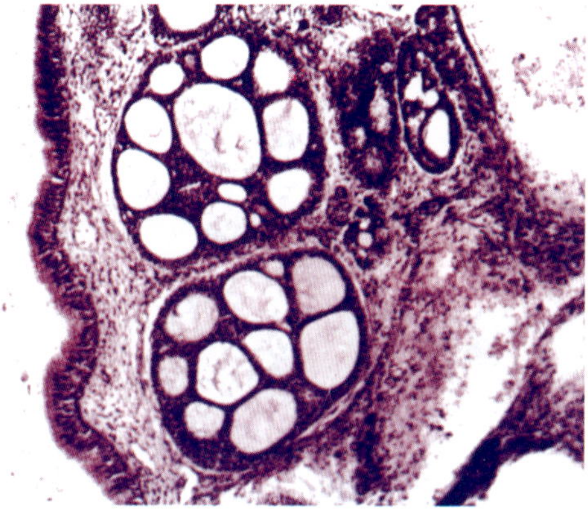

Fig.110 Adenoid cystic carcinoma of nasopharynx (same case as in Fig.108, different field and under high power)

Figure shows:the image of typical cribriform structure of adenoid cystic carcinoma can be seen near mucosal surface. (10×40)

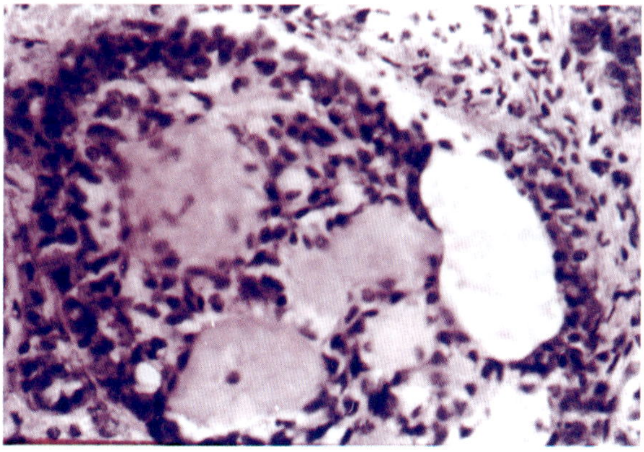

Fig.111 Adenoid cystic carcinoma of nasopharynx (same case as in Fig.108) (10×40)

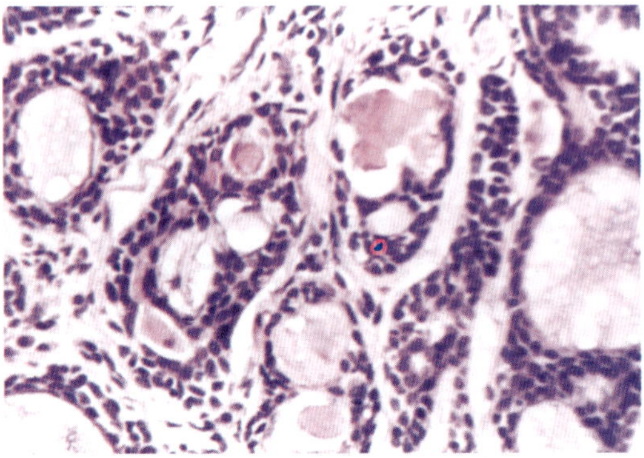

Fig.112 Adenoid cystic carcinoma of nasopharynx (same case as in Fig.108)

Figure shows:pleomorphic features of cancerous glandular structure. (10×40)

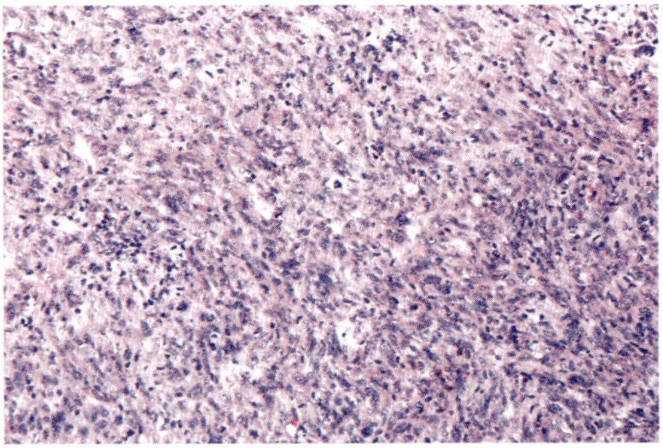

Fig.113 Adenoid cystic carcinoma of nasopharynx after radiotherapy combined with malignant fibrous histiocytoma

Male, 45 years old. In 1970, he had a nasal polypectomy because of nasal obstruction; pathological diagnosis was cylindroma. He recurred after one year, and then received surgery and radiotherapy (1972, 1974, 1977) for three times in some hospital; recently he recurred again and came to receive radical cure.

Figure shows: the tumor contains two main elements: one is primary adenoid cystic carcinoma uncontrolled by radiotherapy;the other contains malignant fibroblasts, malignant histiocytes, polynuclear and giant nuclei tumor cells, which originate from mesenchyme. Phagocytosis of adipoid and blood red cells, as well as hemosiderosis can be seen in these histiocytes. (10×10)

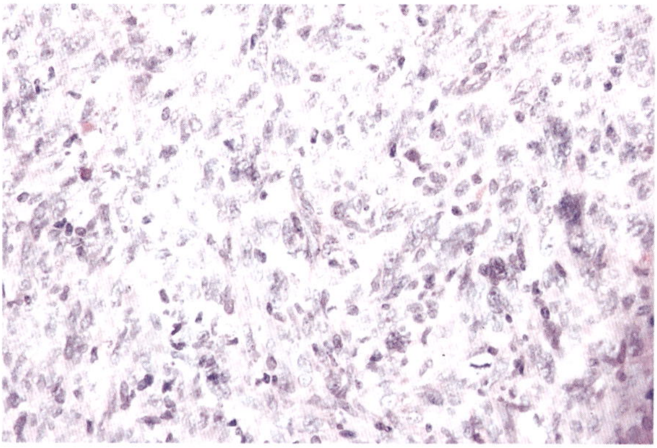

Fig.114 Adenoid cystic carcinoma of nasopharyngeal after radiotherapy combined with malignant fibrous histiocytoma (same case as in Fig.113,under high power) (10×40)

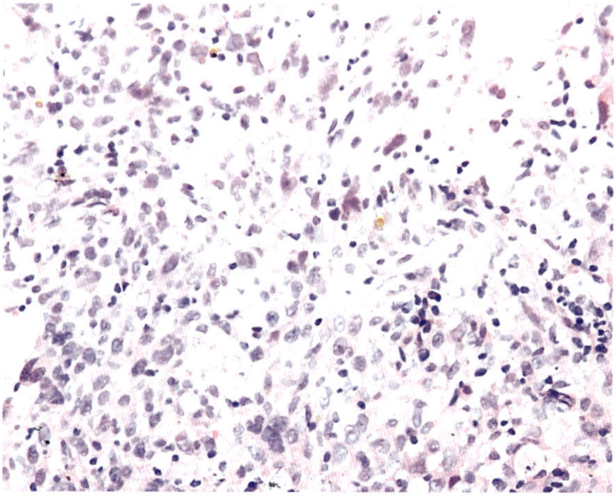

Fig.115 Adenoid cystic carcinoma of nasopharynx complicated with malignant fibrous histiocytoma after radiotherapy (same case as in Fig.114, another field and under high power) (10×40)

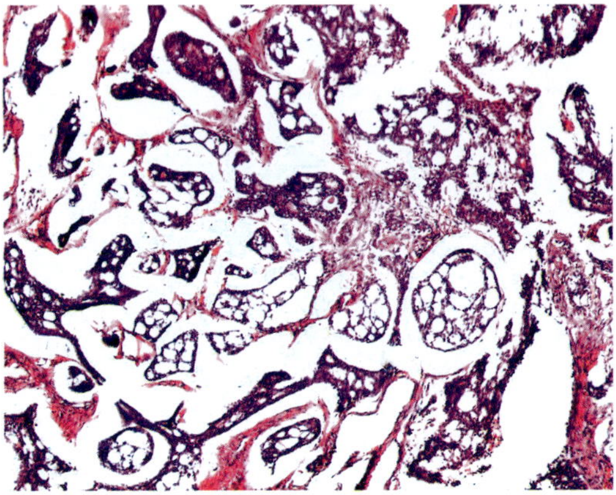

Fig.116 Adenoid cystic carcinoma of nasopharynx complicated with malignant fibrous histiocytoma after radiotherapy (same case as in Fig.115)

Figure shows: the image of primary adenoid cystic carcinoma. (10×10)

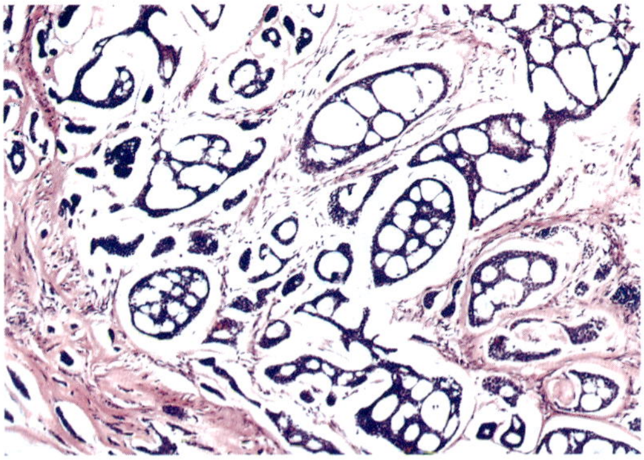

Fig.117 Adenoid cystic carcinoma of nasopharynx complicated with malignant fibrous histiocytoma after radiotherapy (same case as in Fig. 116, different field) (10×10)

4. Benign and malignant tumors originated from mesenchymal tissue in nasopharynx

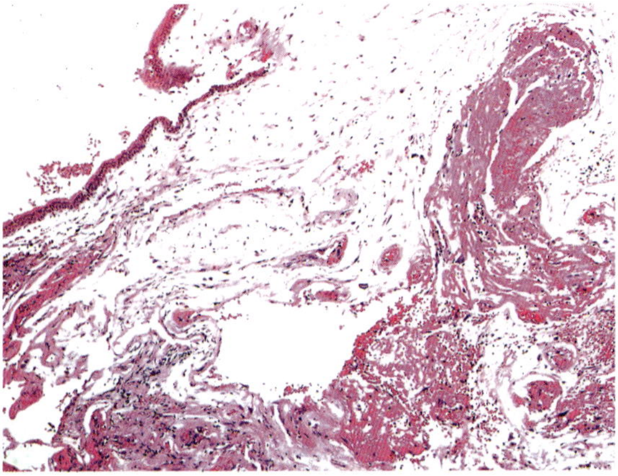

Fig.118 Fibrohemangioma/Angiofibroma of nasopharynx

Male,16 years old.Figure shows: tumor is composed of fibroblasts

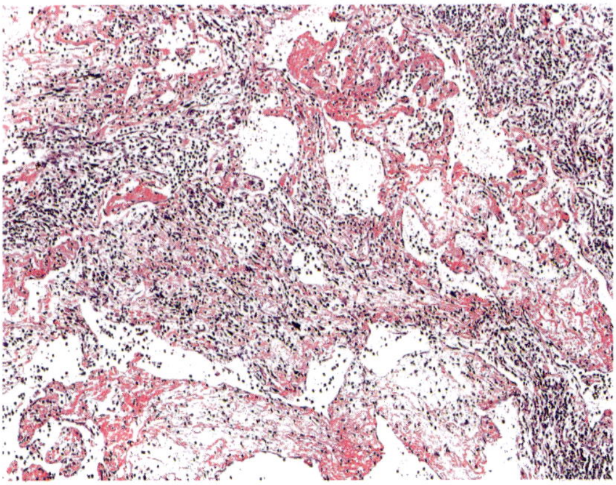

Fig.119 Fibrohemangioma(Angiofibroma) of nasopharynx (same case as in Fig.118, another field)

Figure shows: tumor is composed of cavernous venous sinuses, and there is tumorous fibroblast hyperplasia in stroma. (10×10)

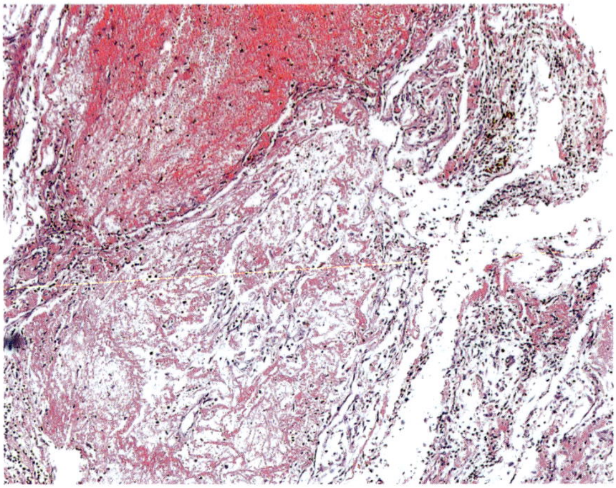

Fig.120 Fibrohemangioma(fibroangioma) of nasopharynx (same case as in Fig.119, another field)

Figure shows: thrombosis in a blood vessel. (10×10)

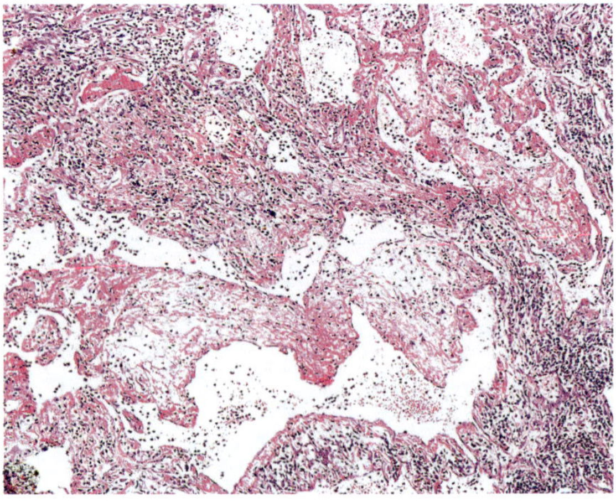

Fig.121 Fibrohemangioma(fibroangioma) of nasopharynx (same case as in Fig. 120, another field) (10×10)

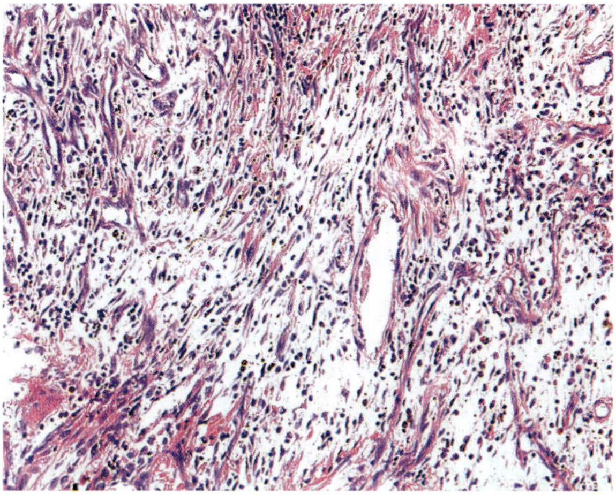

Fig.122 Fibrohemangioma(fibroangioma) of nasopharynx (same case as in Fig.121, under high power)

Figure shows: fibroblasts hypertrophy and hyperplasia. (10×40)

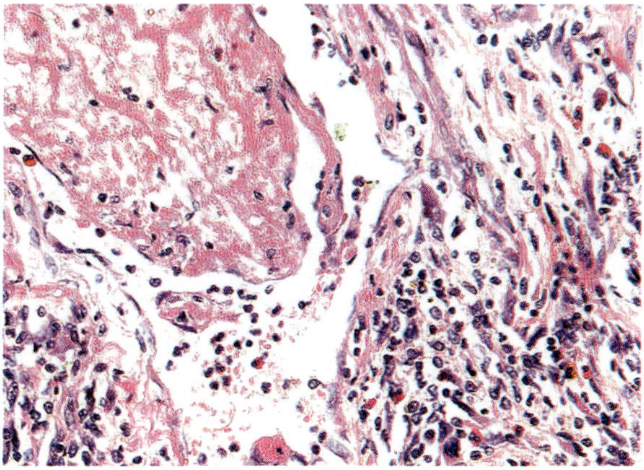

Fig.123 Fibrohemangioma(fibroangioma) of nasopharynx (same case as in Fig.122, another field) (10×40)

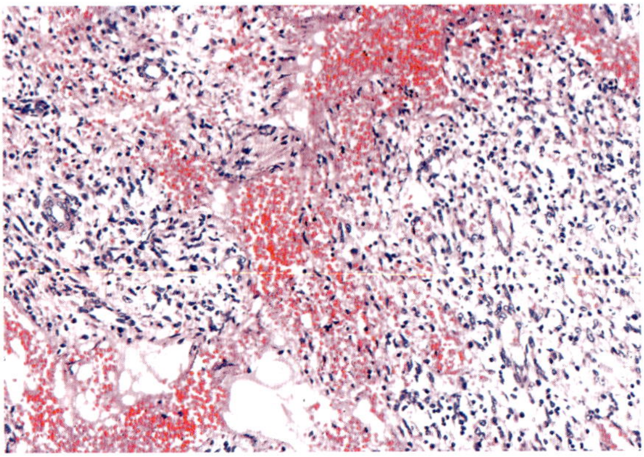

Fig.124 Juvenile fibrohemangioma of nasopharynx

Male,25 years old. He had left nasal obstruction, anemia and severe hemorrhages for ten times more, without tinnitus and headache.

Examination: The neoplasm ($1.2 \times 1.2 \times 1.0 cm^3$) of left parietal nasopharynx extended to left posterior narises and the neoplasm bleeding easily by palpation, with clear border and solid texture. He had a severe hemorrhage at surgery.

Figure shows: the tumor composed of fibrous tissue and blood vessels, and its fibrous tissue active hyperlplasia. Most of all are fibroblasts combined with a few of juvenile stellate cells. (10×10)

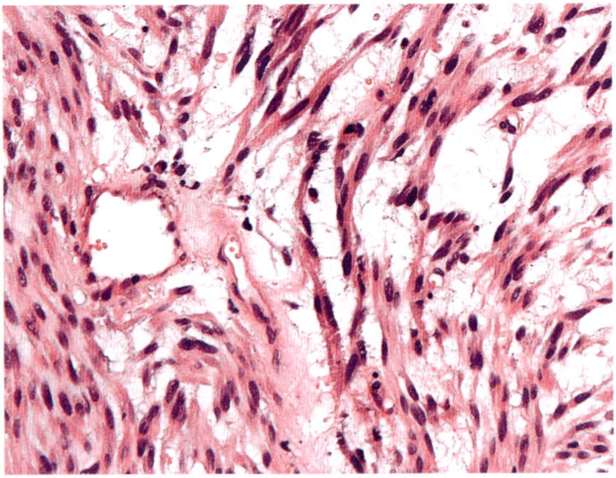

Fig.125 Juvenile fibrohemangioma of nasopharynx (same case as in Fig.124, under high power) (10×40)

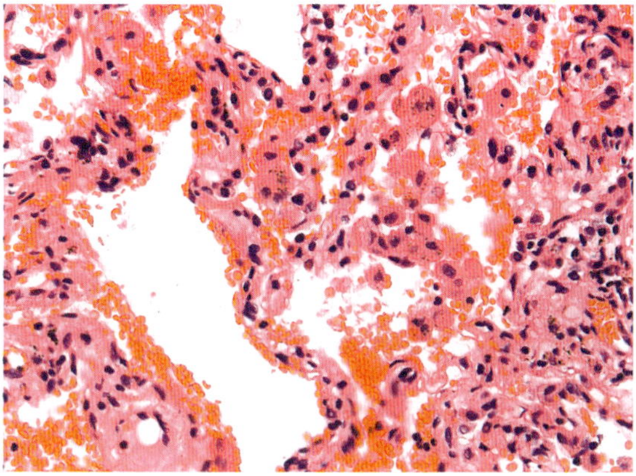

Fig.126 Cavernous hemangioma of nasopharynx

Male, 17 years old. He had nasal obstruction for half a year, the neoplasm of nasopharynx bleeds easily by palpation. Figure shows: lots of cavernous vessels with blood filling up and have only one layer endothelium lining. The blood sinuses are separated by fibrous connective tissue. (10× 40)

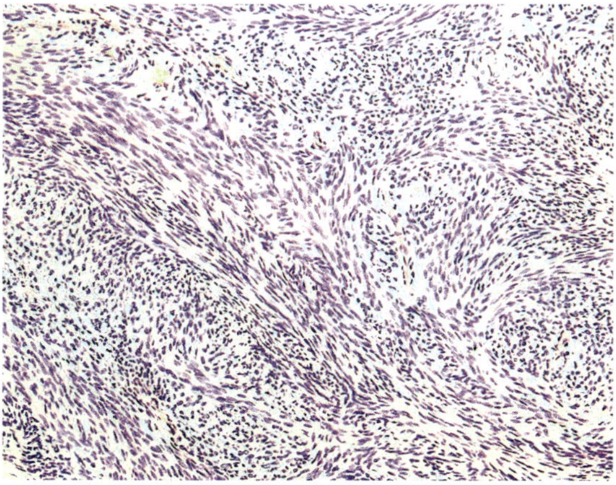

Fig.127 Neurilemmoma of nasopharynx

Male, 52 years old. Figure shows: tumor has intact capsule. Spindle tumor cells have abundant fibers, and the nuclei arrange in palisades. (10× 20)

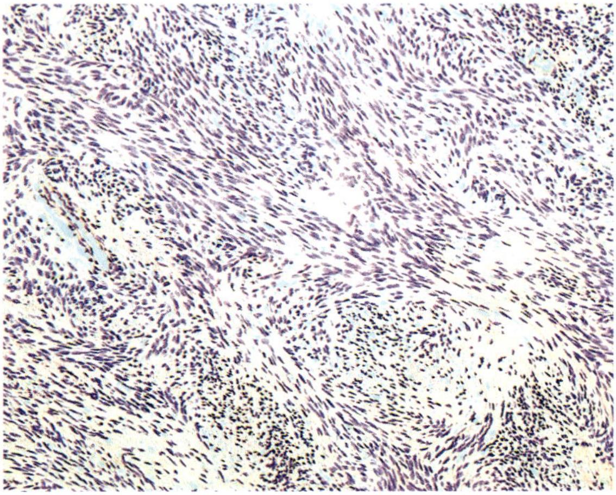

Fig.128 Neurilemmoma of nasopharynx
(same case as in Fig.127,another field) (10×20)

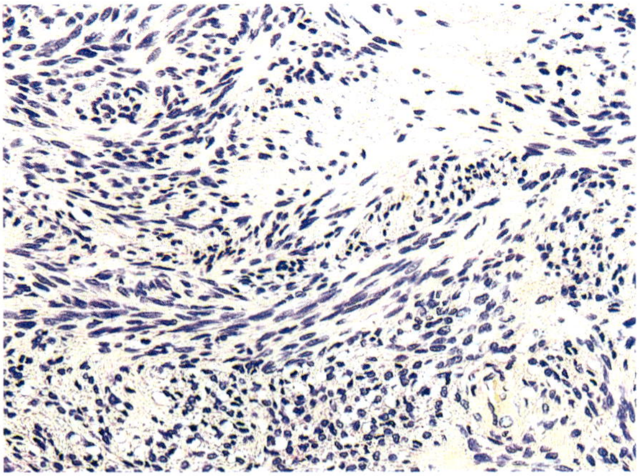

Fig.129 Neurilemmoma of nasopharynx
(same case as in Fig.128, under high power) (10×40)

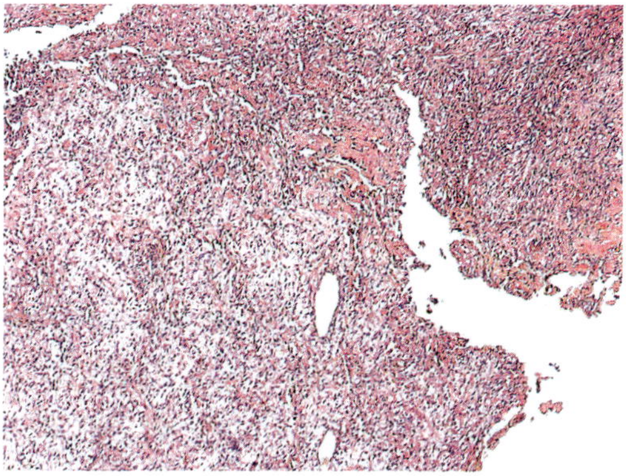

Fig.130 Neurofibroma of nasopharynx

Male, 20 years old. He had the nasophayngeal neoplasm for half a year, without bloody sputum and any other illness.

Clinic examination: A projective neoplasm under nasopharyngeal mucosa of right lateral–wall, with smooth surface, clear capsule and wide basis, extends to pharynx as a giant mass.

Figure shows: there are spindle or stellate tumor cells, with abundant fibers similar to waves and hypochromatic, and their nuclei are small and flexural. Loose stroma is edematous, combined with mucoid degenaretion. The tumor has no obvious capsule. (10×10)

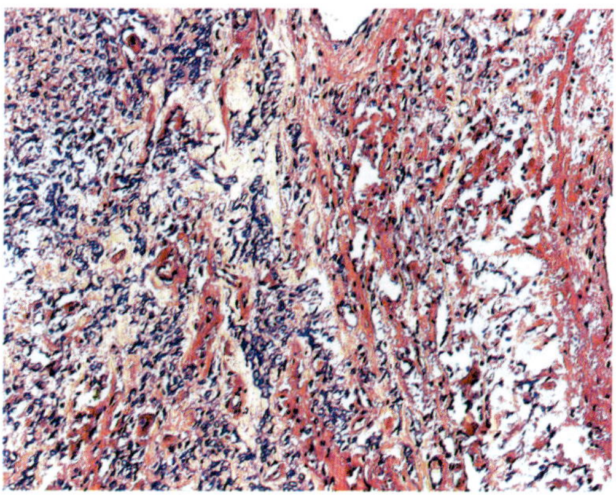

Fig.131 Neurofibroma of nasopharynx
(same case as in Fig.130, under high power) (10×40)

Figure shows: tumor cells with loose structures arrange in irregular palisades.

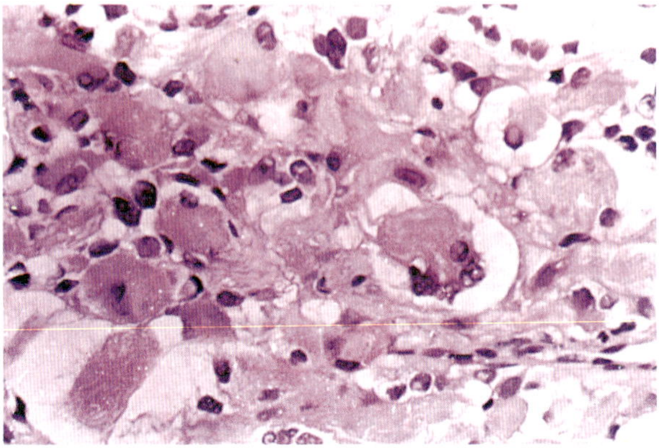

Fig.132 Pleomorphic rhadomyosarcoma of nasopharynx

Female, 68 years old. Figure shows: the tumor is composed of pleomorphic rhadomyoblasts with mononucleus and polynuclei. The tumor cells are with abundant cytoplasm and strong eosinophilic staining. Vertical myofibril can be seen, and cross striation can be found occasionly. The existence of cross striation can be confirmed by phosphotungstic acid hematoxylin stain. (10×40)

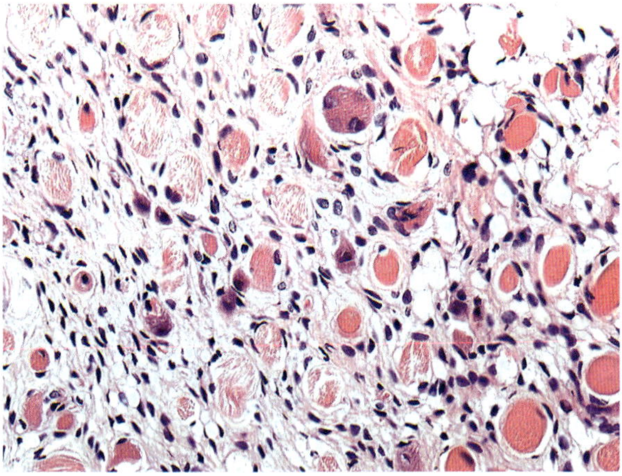

Fig.133 Pleomorphic rhadomyosarcoma of nasopharynx (same case as in Fig.132, another field)

Figure shows: pleomorphic rhadomyosarcoma cells with irregular arrangement and pleomorphism. (10×40)

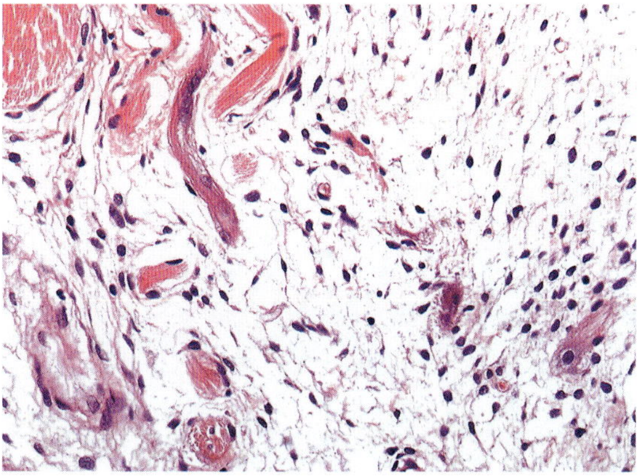

Fig.134 Pleomorphic rhadomyosarcoma of nasopharynx (same case as in Fig. 133, another field)

Figure shows: different shapes of tumor cells, such as ribbon, spindle, hand-mirror-like and spider-like. Parts of them have vesicular cytoplasm. (10×40)

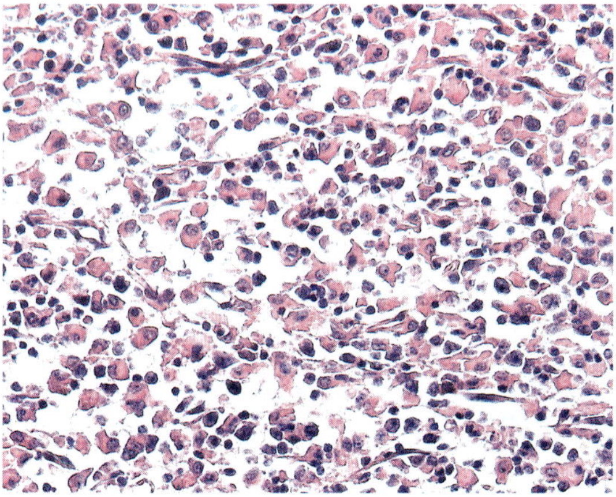

Fig.135 Rhadomyosarcoma of nasopharynx, embryonic type

Female, 6 years old. The necrotic neoplasm can be seen in nasopharynx. Figure shows:most of tumor cells, with diffuse distribution,are small round and undifferentiated rhadomyoblasts; a few of rich cytoplasm strong eosinophilic and relative well-differentiated rhadomyoblasts also can be seen. (10×40)

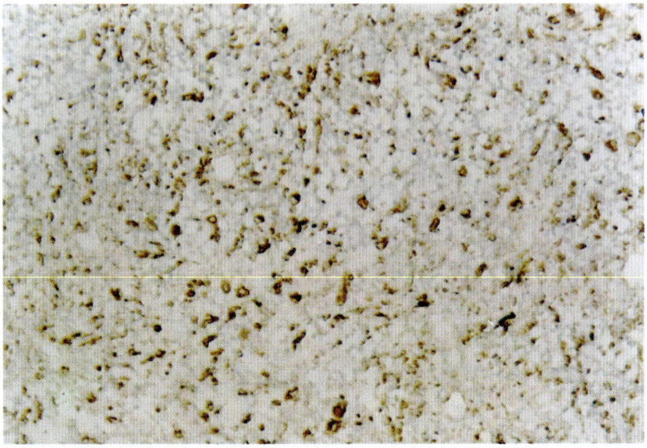

Fig.136 Rhadomyosarcoma of nasopharynx, embryonic type (same case as in Fig.135 immunochemistry staining)(10×20)

Immunohistochemistry: Actin(HHF35) (+)

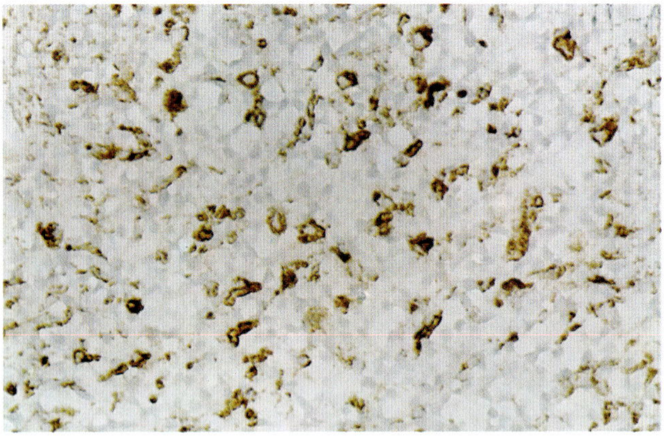

Fig.137 Rhadomyosarcoma of nasopharynx, embryonic type (same case as in Fig.136, under high power) (10×40)

Immunohistochemistry: Actin(HHF35) (+)

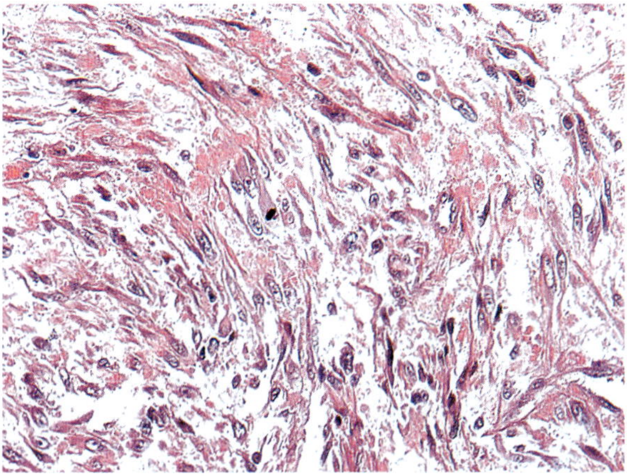

Fig.138 Leiomyosarcoma of nasopharynx

Female, 24 years old. She had bloody nasal secretion in the morning for two months.

Examination: the pink and projective neoplasm of nasopharyngel fossa could be seen, and the neoplasm bleeds easily by palpation.

Figure shows: wide-spindle tumor cells with obtuse two-ends of nuclei and eosinophilic cytoplasm. A few of tumor cells are slight atypical. Mitoses can be seen in figure. (10×40)

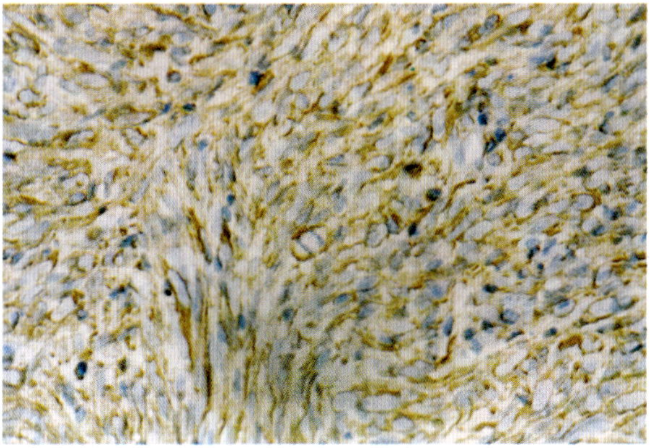

Fig.139 Leiomyosarcoma of nasopharynx (same case as in Fig. 138, SMA test)

Immunohistochemistry: Actin (smooth muscle) (+) (10×40)

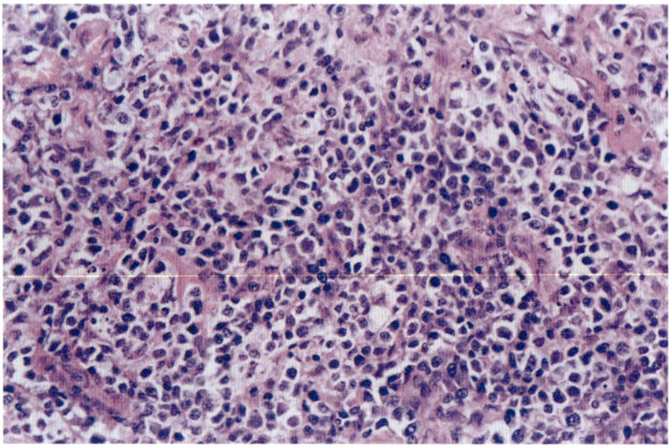

Fig.140 Non-Hodgkin's lymphoma(NHL) of nasopharynx

Figure shows: the tumor is composed of uniformed small-round lyphmocytes, which distribute diffusely. (10×40)

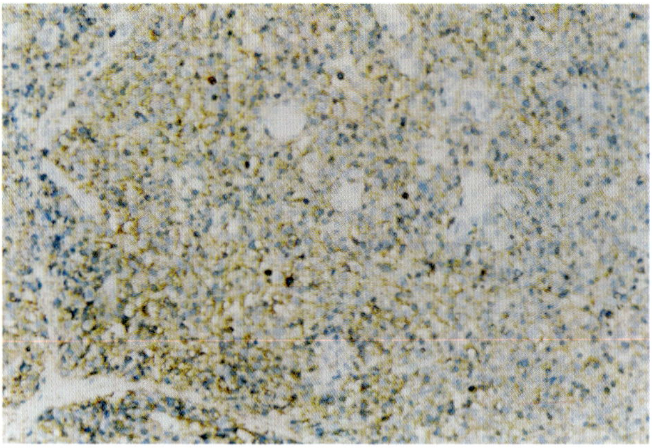

Fig.141 Non-Hodgkin's lymphoma(NHL) of nasopharynx (same case as in Fig.140 LCA test)(10×40)

Immunohistochemistry: LCA (+)

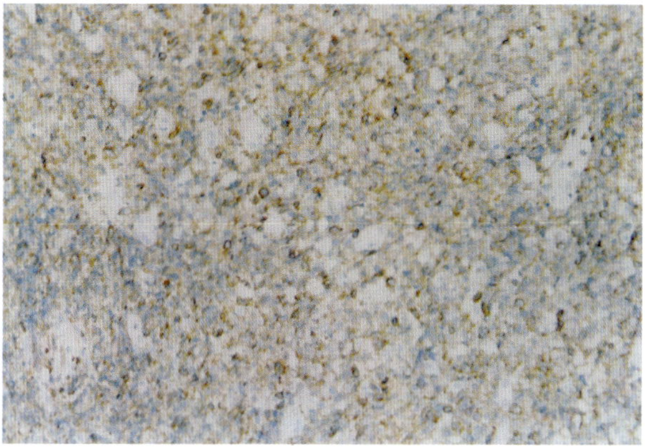

Fig.142 Non-Hodgkin's lymphoma(NHL) of nasopharynx (same case as in Fig.140 CD45RO test)

Immunohistochemistry:CD45RO(+)(10×40)

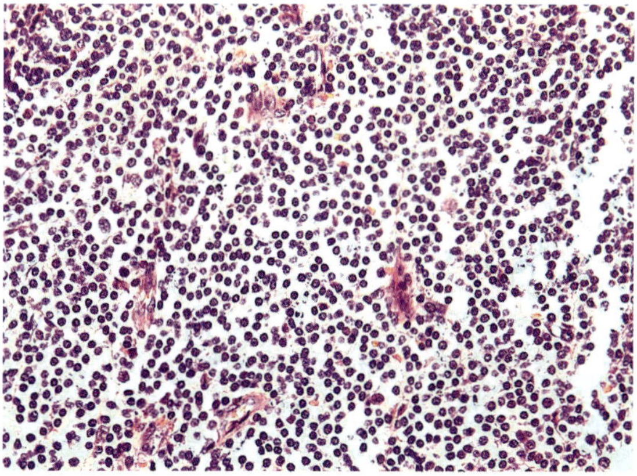

Fig.143 Non-Hodgkin's lymphoma(NHL) of nasopharynx (same case as in Fig.140, another field)

Figure shows: the small and round tumor cells possess homogeneous nuclear chromatin and scanty cytoplasm, no nucleoli. (10×40) This case was confirmed as T cell lymphoma by CD45RO test. (same case as in Figure shows:pleomorphic features of cancerous glandular structure. (10×40)

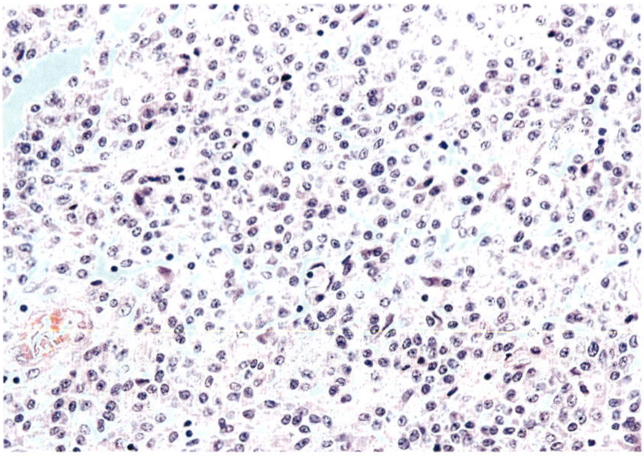

Fig.144 Non-Hodgkin's lymphoma(NHL) of nasopharynx

Female, 74 years old. Figure shows: the tumor cells are diffuse, distributed around vessels, with moderate cytoplasm, varying size, hyperchromatic nuclei, and asymmetry nuclei which are similar as nuclei of plasma cells. Part of them has nucleoli. Morphological diagnosis is lymphoplasmacytic lpymphoma. (10×40)

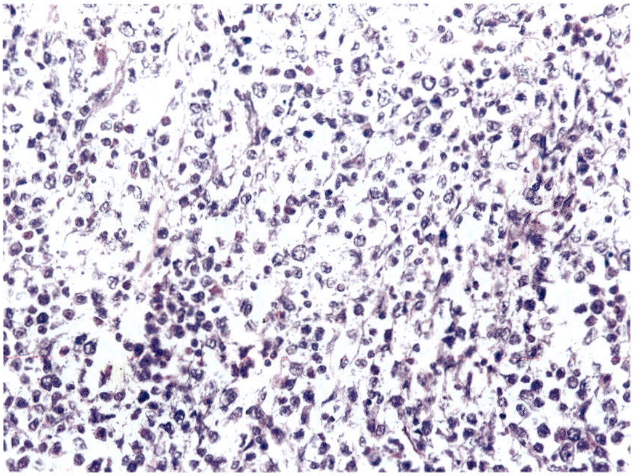

Fig.145 Non-Hodgkin's lymphorna (NHL) of nasopharynx accompanied with lymphoma of stomach

Male, 47 years old. Figure shows: irregular round tumor cell, with visible nuclei and loose , granular chromatin, as well as lilac and clear cytoplasm distribute diffusely. (10×40)

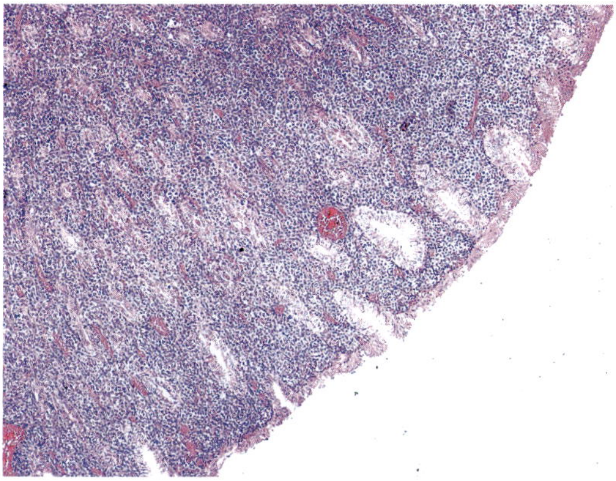

Fig.146 Non-Hodgkin's lymphorna (NHL) of nasopharynx accompanied with lymphoma of stomach (same case as in Fig.145)

The slides were made by the gastrectomy sample of the patient's stomach tumor. (10×10)

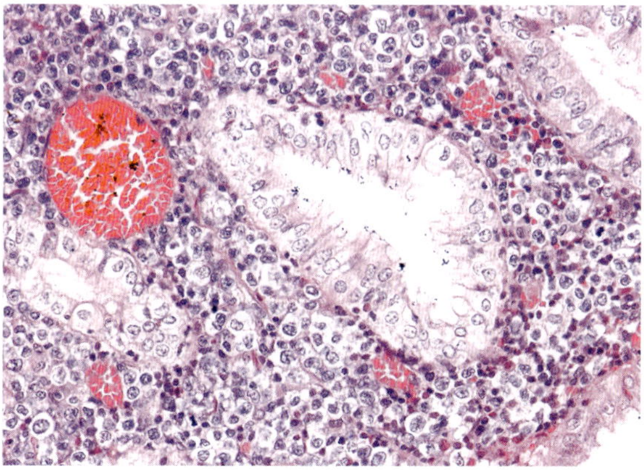

Fig.147 Non–Hodgkin's lymphorna (NHL) of nasopharynx accompanied with lymphoma of stomach (same case as in Fig.146, under high power)

Figure shows: diffuse lymphoid tumor cells distribute among gastric mucosal glands, and their morphosis are similar to that of Fig.145 (10×40)

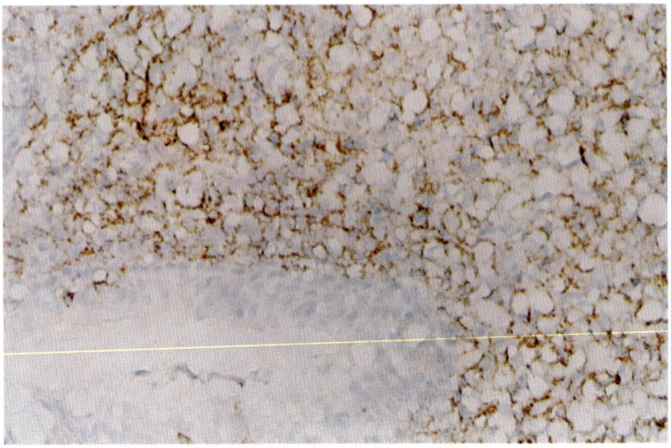

Fig.148 Non-Hodgkin's lymphorna (NHL) of nasopharynx accompanied with lym-phoma of stomach (same case as in Fig.147, Immunohistochemistry)

Immunohistochemistry: CD20 (+) (10×40)

Figure shows: B cells of CD20 positive diffusely infiltrate in nasopharygeal and stomach tissue.

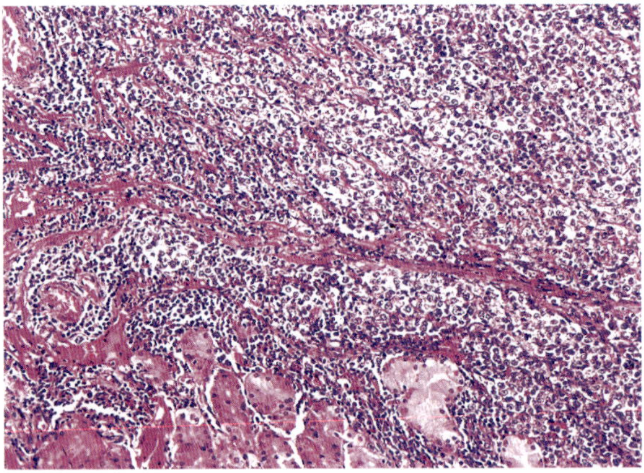

Fig.149 Non-Hodgkin's lymphorna (NHL) of nasopharynx accompanied with lymphoma of stomach (same case as in Fig.148)

Figure shows: lymphoma cells diffusely infiltrate in gastric submucosa and muscularis, whose morphosis are similar to that of Fig.147. It can't be sure yet that the primary focus is stomach or nasopharynx or both, namely polycentric originations. (10×10)

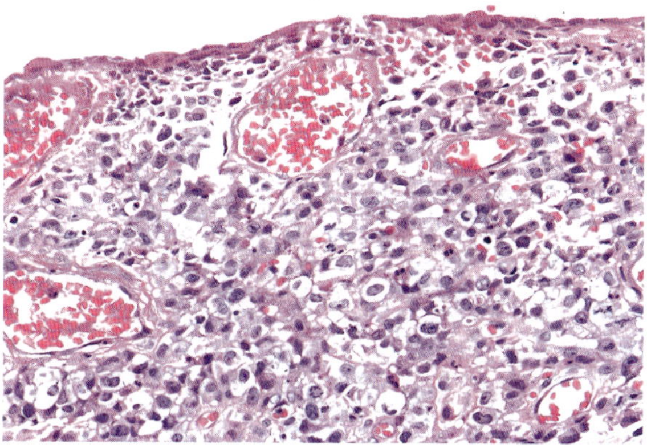

Fig.150 Non-Hodgkin's lymphoma(NHL) of nasopharynx (flexuous nuclear type)

Male, 9 years old. Figure shows: squamous epithelia of the tumor surface are intact. Diffuse and irregular lymphoma cells invade lamina propria. (10×40)

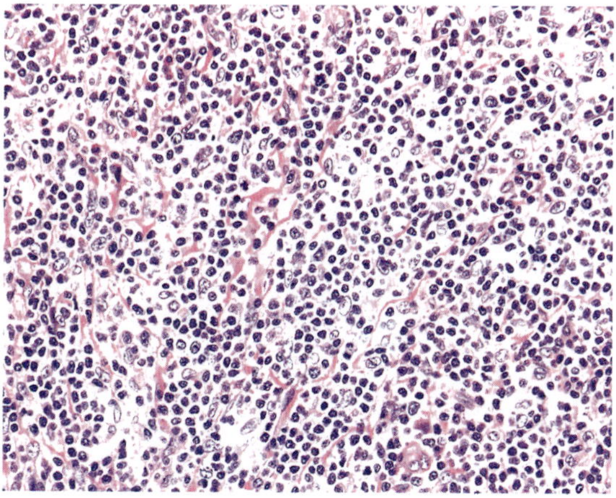

Fig.151 Non-Hodgkin's lymphoma(NHL) of nasopharynx (same case as in Fig.150)

Figure shows: round tumor cells with varying size (3-10μm) and scanty cytoplasm. Nclear morphosis is the base of diagnosis, shallow and deep grooves can be seen in the nuclear surfaces, sometimes neclear shape is like "chicken-claw" with homogeneous nuclear chromatin. Immunohistochemistry, they originate from T cells. (10×20)

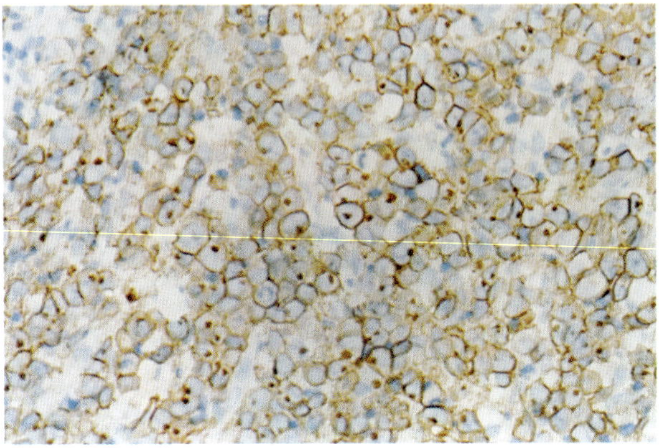

Fig.152 Non-Hodgkin's lymphoma(NHL) of nasopharynx (same case as in Fig.151, Immunohistochemistry) (10×40)

Immunohistochemistry: CD30 (+)

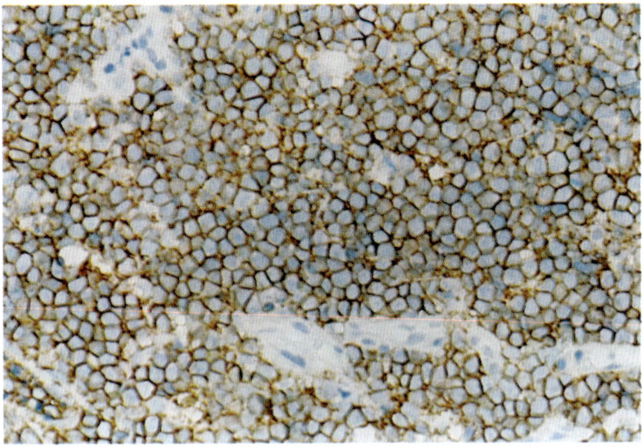

Fig.153 Non-Hodgkin's lymphoma(NHL) of nasopharynx (T-cell lymphoma) (10×20)

Immunohistochemistry: CD45RO (+)

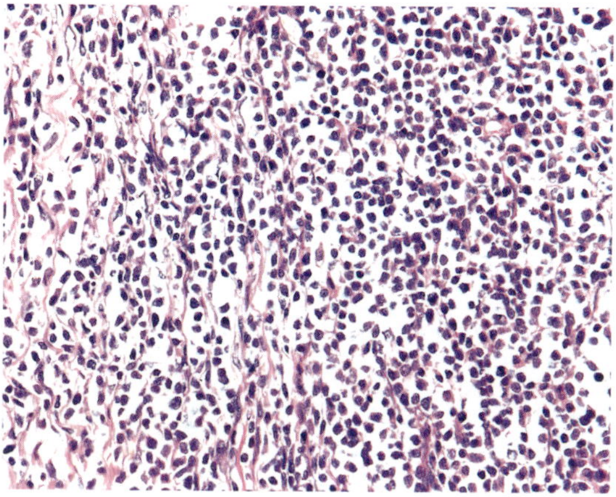

Fig.154 Non-Hodgkin's lymphoma(NHL) of nasopharynx (same case as in Fig.151, another field) (10×20)

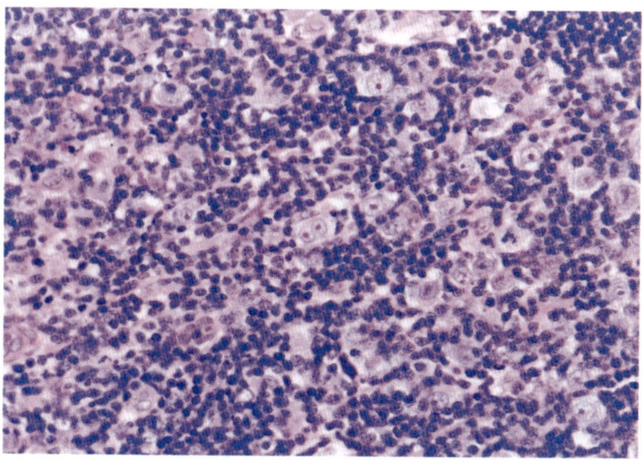

Fig.155 Hodgkin's lymphoma of nasopharynx (lymphocyte predominance type)

Female, 35 years old. She had lymphatic lumps of bilateral neck, nasal obstruction and intermittently long-term low fever without any cause. She had no headache and tinnitus.The neoplasm of nasopharynx could be seen by pharyngorhinoscopy.Figure shows: nasopharyngeal lymph tissue active hyperplasia. Reed-sternberg cells (R-S cell) can be found occasionally. (a Hodgkin's cell, in the middle of figure) (10×20)

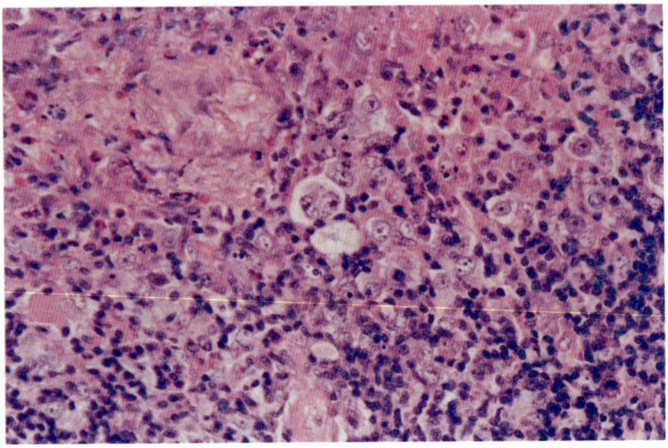

Fig.156 Hodgkin's lymphoma of nasopharynx
(same case as in Fig.155) (10×40)

Figure shows: the structure of the Reed-sternberg cell (R-S cell) is clearer in the middle of figure. (10×40)

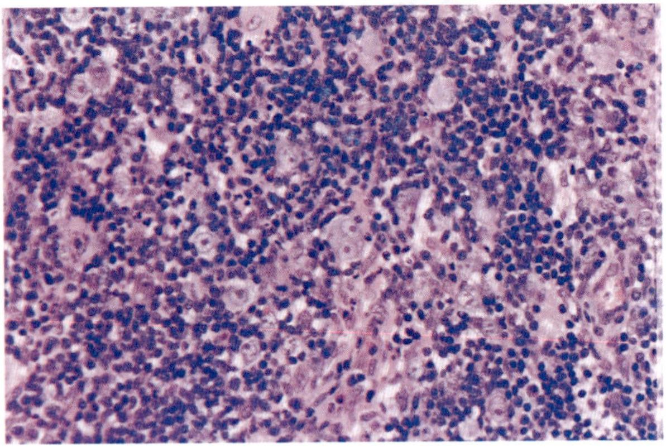

Fig.157 Hodgkin's lymphoma of nasopharynx
(same as Fig.155,the lesions of jugular lymph nodes and nasopharynx are same)

Figure shows: the structure of Reed-sternberg cell (R-S cell) is more typical in the middle of figure. (10×10)

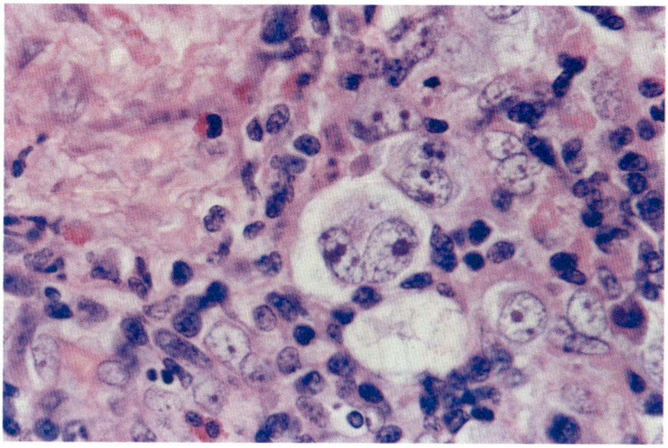

Fig.158 Hodgkin's lymphoma of nasopharynx
(same case as in Fig.157,under oil lens) (10×100)

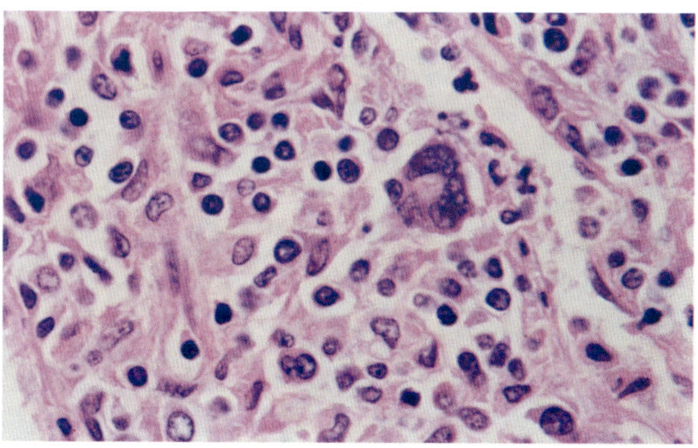

Fig.159 Hodgkin's lymphoma of nasopharynx
(same case as in Fig.158,different field)

Figure shows: polynuclear Reed-sternberg cell (R-S cell) can be found in the middle of figure.(10×100)

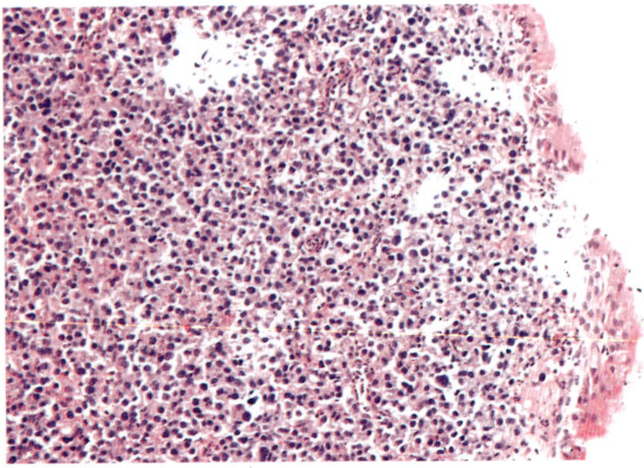

Fig.160 Plasmacytoma of nasopharynx

Male, 34 years old. He had intermittently nasal hemorrhage for one year more, and had a severe hemorrhage ten days ago.

Clinic examination: The neoplasm ($1.5\times1.2\times1.0cm^3$) of nasopharynx could be seen, with erosional surface and a little of gore.

Figure shows: nasophayngeal mocusa has been atrophy. The tumor locate in lamina propria, and protrudes mucosa projected as a polyp. Uniform tumor cells have abundant cytoplasm. Most of hyperchromatic and round nuclei are side placement. Immature tumorous plasma cells are larger, which have larger and centrally placed nuclei and sometimes binuclear and giant nuclear tumor cells can be found. (10×10)

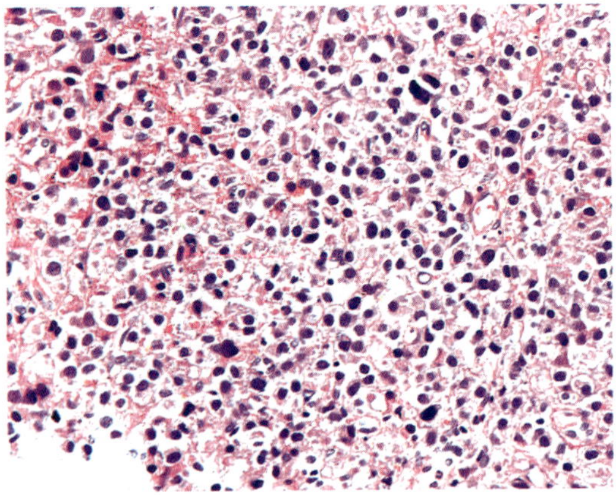

Fig.161 Plasmacytoma of nasopharynx (same case as in Fig.160) (10×40)

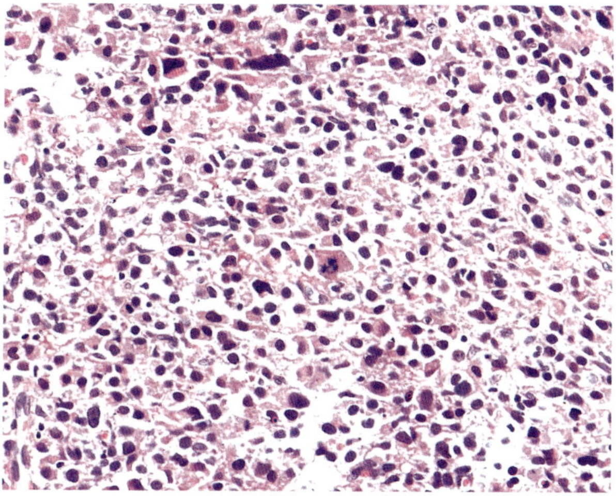

Fig.162 Plasmacytoma of nasopharynx
(same case as in Fig.161) (10×40)

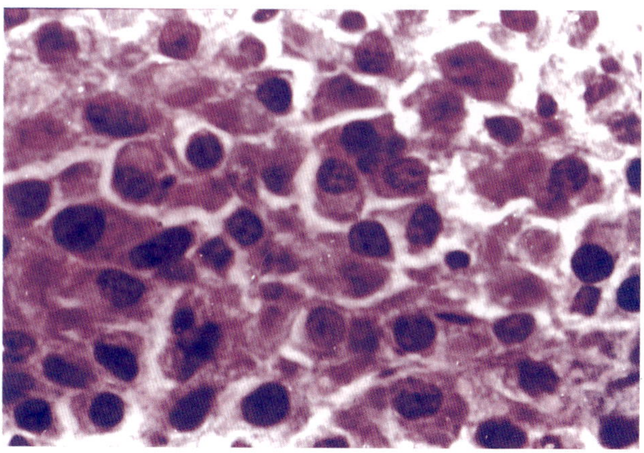

Fig.163 Plasmacytoma of nasopharynx
(same case as in Fig.162,another field) (10×100)

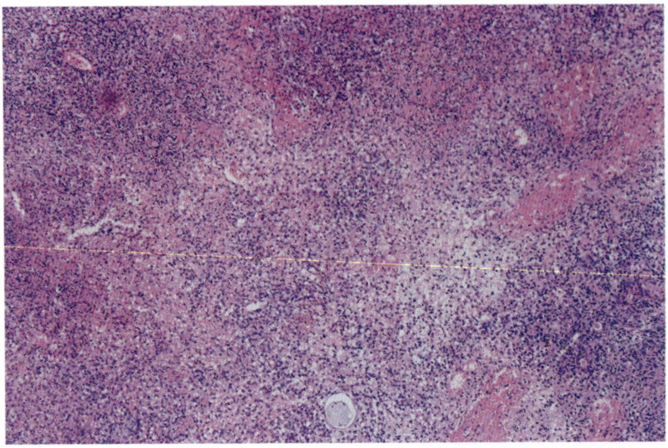

Fig.164 Clinical sign as necrosis granuloma of nasopharynx (NK/T-lymphoma)

Male, 37 years old. Figure shows: there is a mass of necrotic tissue, the vascular walls are necrotic also and a few of the atypical tumor cells left among them. (10×10)

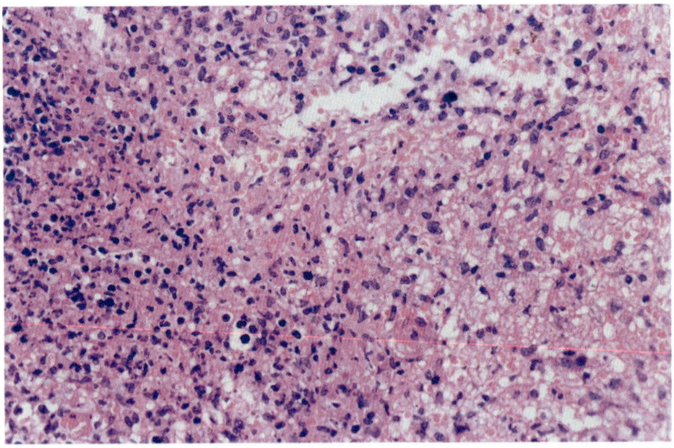

Fig.165 Clinical findings suspicious of gangrenous granuloma of nasopharynx (NK/T-lymphoma) (same case as in Fig.164, under high power)

Figure shows: the tumor cells are with varying size and anaplasia. Mitoses can be seen in the figure.(10×40)

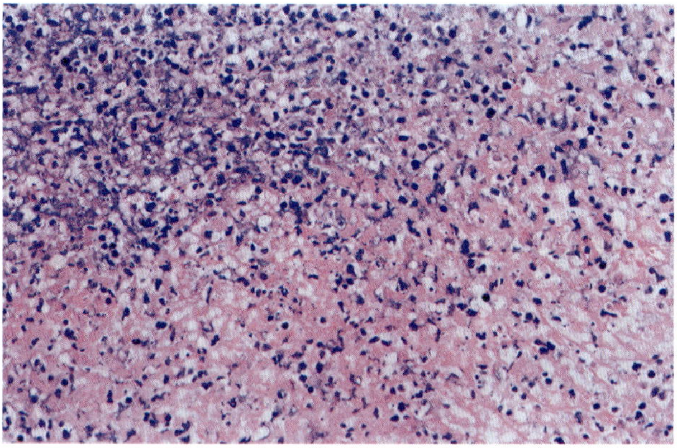

Fig.166 Clinical findings suspicious of gangrenous granuloma of nasopharynx (NK/T-lymphoma)

Male, 29 years old. Figure shows: the tissue necrosis and blurry structure. A few of atypical nuclei of tumor cells can be seen. (10×40)

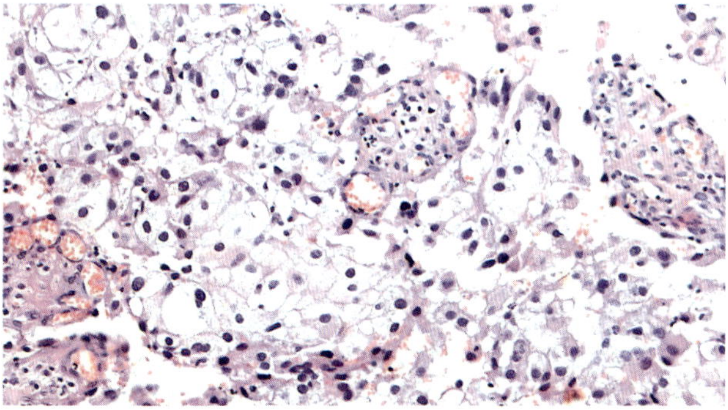

Fig.167 Chondroma of nasopharynx

Male, 40 years old. He had tinnitus, hypoacusis, and left facial hypoesthesia. radiograph indicated: sphenoid bone was destroyed.There is a graywhite and semi-transparent nasopharyngeal tumor which has no intact capsule with the gelatinous section.

Figure shows: the tumor cells have varying size and irregular arrangement. Cytoplasm contains lots of mucus or presents as giant vacuoles. Round or oval nuclei are small, and hyperchromatic. The nuclei locate centrally or a side extruded by mucus, similar to signet-ring cell.(The patient's symptoms indicated cranial nerves were involved.) (10×40)

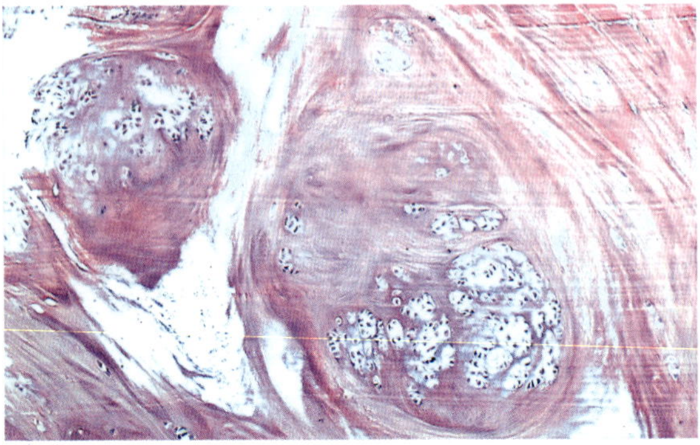

Fig.168 Chondroma of nasopharynx

Male, 34 years old. He had felt pharynx uncomfortable and eyewinker -sense for half a year. There was the neoplasm of posterior-wall of pharynx ($1\times1\times1cm^3$), with slightly projecting and clear border.

Figure shows: the tumor cells are chondrocytes with blue and hyaline cartilage matrix. Chondrocytes, with small and hyperchromatic nuclei, that are larger and more irregular than normal ones, and binuclear cells can be seen occasionally. The tumor may originate from heterotopic chondrocyte nests. (10×10)

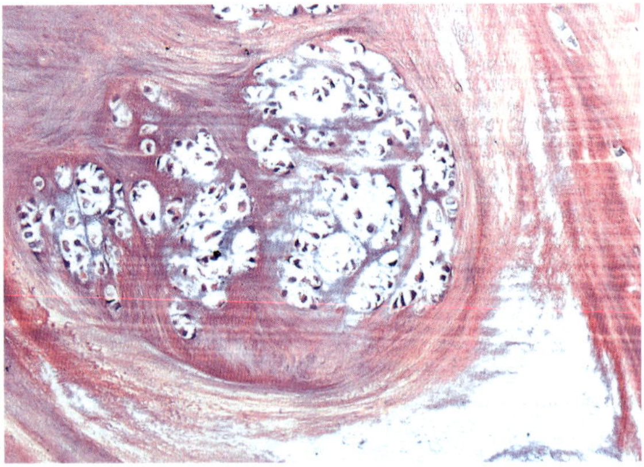

Fig.169 Chondroma of nasopharynx
(same case as in Fig.168,under high power) (10×40)

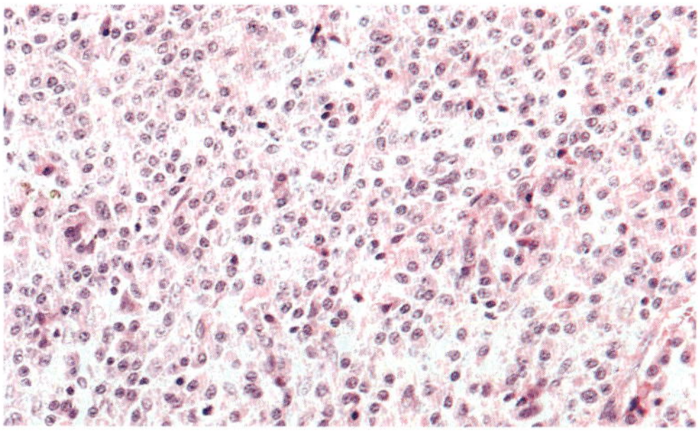

Fig.170 Acidophilic (or oxyphilic) cell adenoma of nasopharynx

Female, 63 years old.She had felt nasal obstruction for four years more, and then recured radiotherapy and chemical therapy; but the neoplasm didn't disappeared completely yet.Two years later, she received radiotherapy again because of nasal obstruction aggravating and the neoplasm enlarging, but the results were not good. She had sickened for seven years,but had no jugular metastasis and cranial nerves involved.

Figure shows: the uniform tumor cells, with small and centrally placed nuclei, , abundant cytoplasm, eosinophilic granules, and no mitosis , arrange in glandular and rosette-like structures. (10×40)

5. Tumors and other diseases of nose

Fig.171–205: Tumors and other diseases of nose

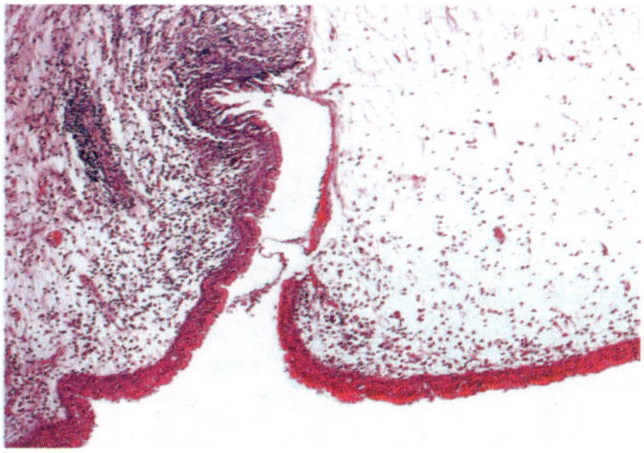

Fig.171 Nasal polyp

Male, 36 years old. He felt nasal obstruction for ten years. Several pinkish-grey, red, with smooth surface polyps could be seen in right narises. Figure shows: polyps are covered by pseudostratified ciliated columnar epithelia with obvious edema under epithelia, and there are some plasma cells, lymphocytes and a few of neutrophil and eosinophil infiltration. (10×10)

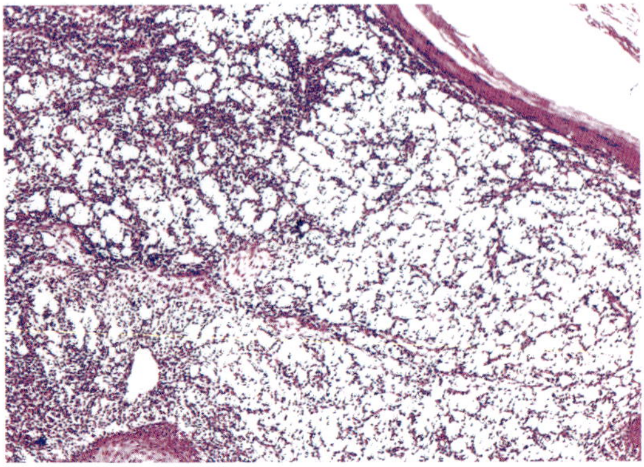

Fig.172 Rhinoscleroma (granulomatous stage)

Male, 35 years old. He had felt nasal obstruction for three years more, and his biopsy was diagnosed as malignant granuloma in another hospital. Then he went to the Tumor Hospital of Sun Yat-sen university,and his biopsy was diagnosed as rhinoscleroma.He has been mended after treatment according to rhinoscleroma.

Figure shows: inflammatory is granuloma composed of lots of foamy cells, plasma cells and inflammatory granular tissue infiltrated by a few of acidophilic leukocytes. Big foamy macrophages, with large volume (Dia. 18-55μm), are round, and are named from cytoplasm filled with vacuoles with varying size. Round or oval and hyperchromatic nuclei place centrally or aside. (10×10)

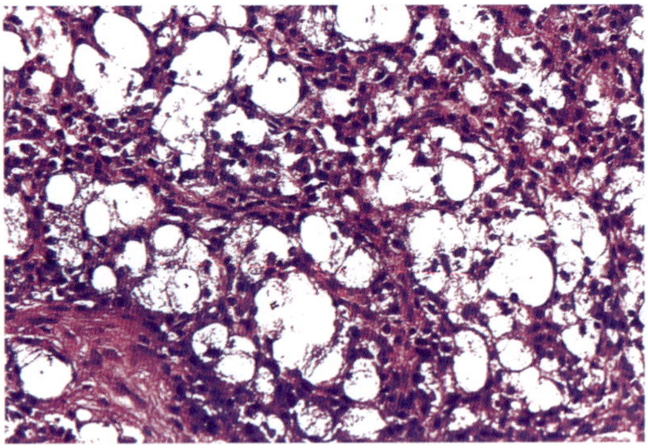

Fig.173 Rhinoscleroma (granulomatous stage) (same case as in Fig.172)

Figure shows: the foamy cytoplasm of rhinoscleroma is vesicular under oil lens. (10×40)

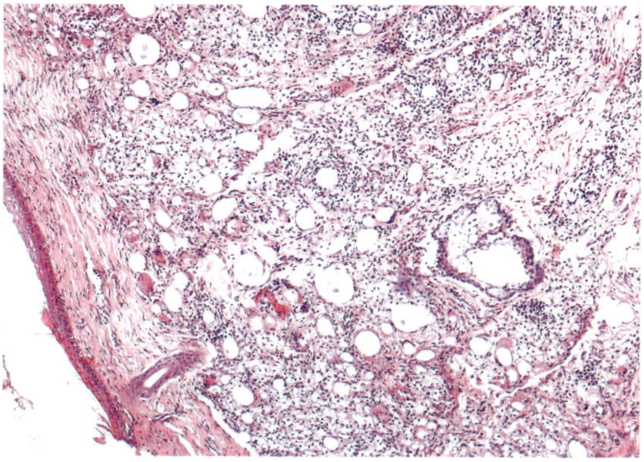

Fig.174 Lepromatous leprosy of nasal septum

Male, 36 years old. He felt nasal obstruction and sniveled for one year more. There is a neoplasm with erosional surface in nasal septum. The nasal septum is perforated and discovered by the bougie.

Figure shows: lepromatous granulomatous neoplasm in nasal septum mucosa is composed of lots of foamy macrophages (lepra cells), lymphocytes, histocytes and plasma cells, especially forming typical leproma, which are big and round, containing mucous materials. Large numbers of red mycobacterium leprae (leprosy bacilli) are demonstrated by acid-fast stain in leprae cells. (10×10)

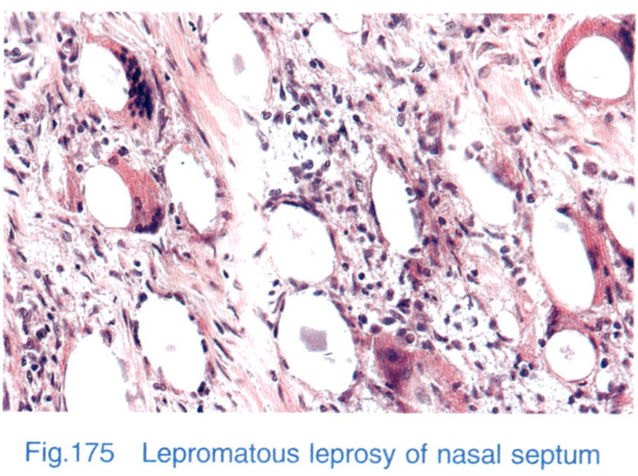

Fig.175 Lepromatous leprosy of nasal septum (same case as in Fig.174, under high power)

Figure shows: lepromas are big and round , containing mucous materials and leprosy bacilli. (10×40)

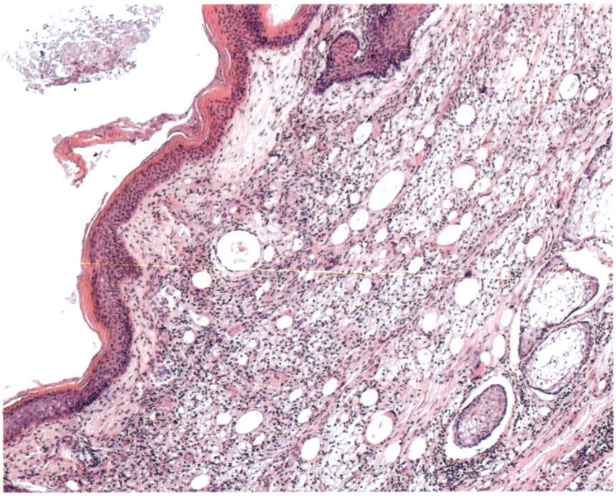

Fig.176 Lepromatous leprosy of nasal septum (acidfast stain) (same case as in Fig.174, another field)

Figure shows: large numbers of red mycobacterium leprae (leprosy bacilli) can be seen in lepromas and foamy macrophages by acid-fast stain (10×10)

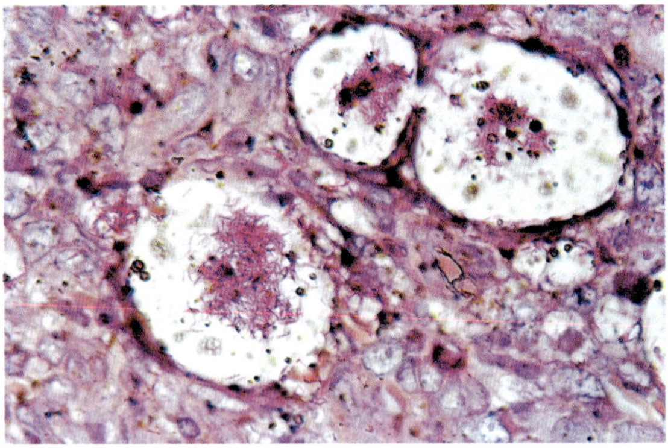

Fig.177 Lepromatous leprosy of nasal septum (same case as in Fig.176, different field of acid-fast stain under oil lens)

Figure shows: large numbers of red mycobacterium leprae (leprosy bacilli) can be seen in lepromas and foamy macrophages by acid-fast stain (10×100)

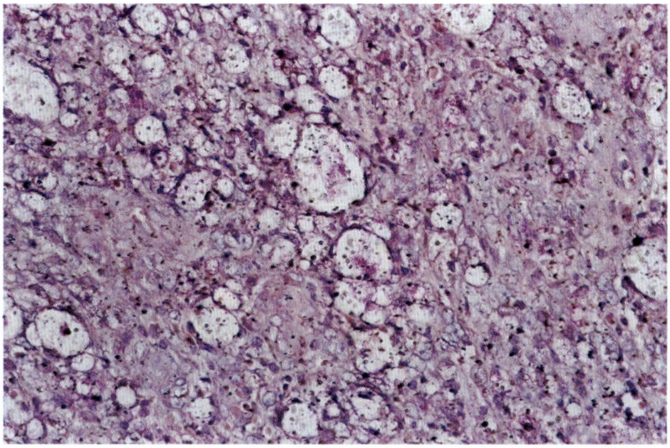

Fig.178 Lepromatous leprosy of nasal septum (same case as in Fig.177, another field)(10×40)

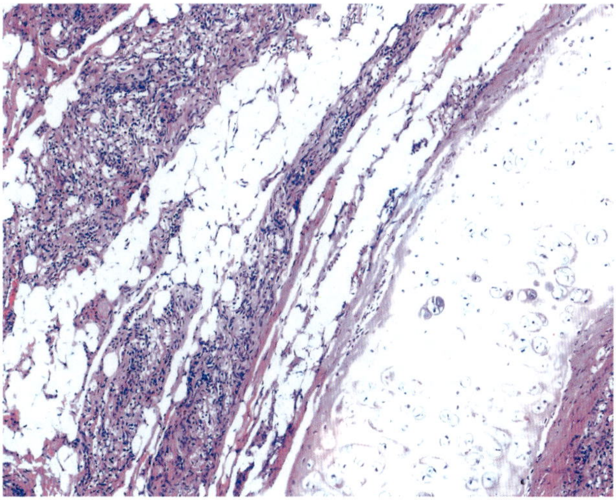

Fig.179 Lepromatous leprosy of nasal septum (same case as in Fig.174,another field)

Figure shows: lepromatous granular tissue hyperplasia in soft tissue near the hyaline cartilage of nasal spetum. (10×10)

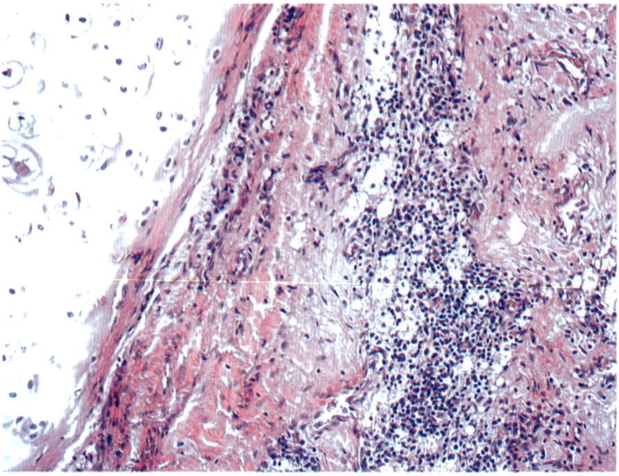

Fig.180 Lepromatous leprosy of nasal septum
(same case as in Fig.162,under high power)

Figure shows: the lesion focus in perichondrium made by a pile of lepromatous leprosy. (10×20)

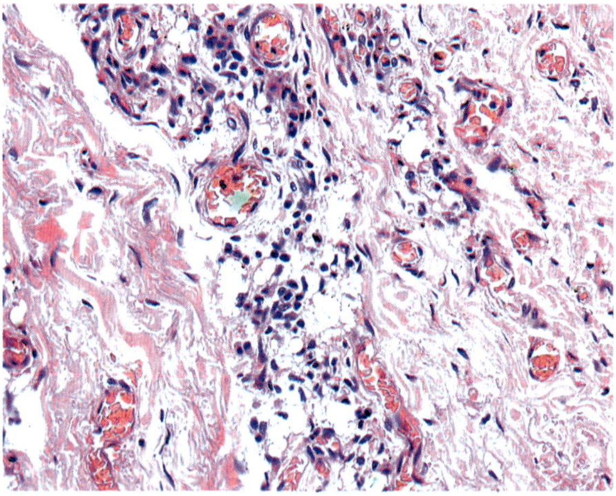

Fig.181 Lepromatous leprosy of nasal septum

Male, 79 years old. He had felt limbs paralysis and edema for three years.

Figure shows: lots of foamy macrophages in leprosy focus near blood vessels. (10×40)

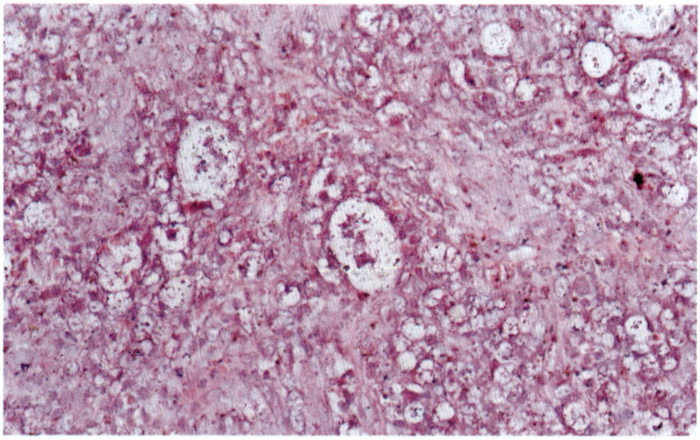

Fig.182 Leprosy of nasal mucosa

Male, adult. Figure shows: Before treatment, large numbers of thick and red mycobacterium leprae (leprosy bacilli) can be seen in lepromatous leprosy of nose and pile in foamy macrophages by acid-fast stain (10×40)

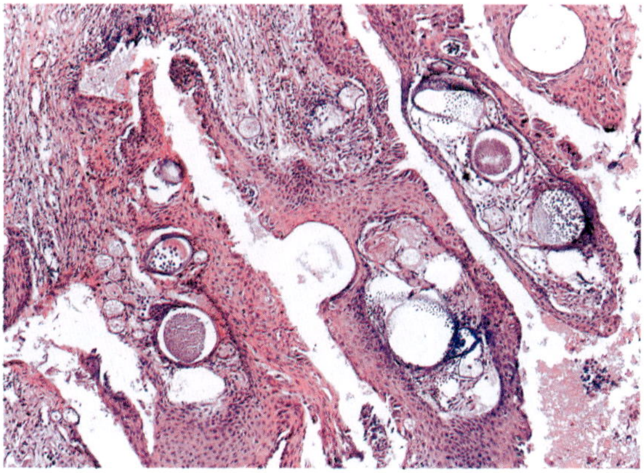

Fig.183 Coccidioidomyocosis (coccidoidal granuloma) of nose

Male, 26 years old. He had the polypoid neoplasm of right inferior nasal conchae for seven years, and recurred after surgery.

Figure shows:squamous epithelia of nasal conchae mucusa papillary are hyperplasia.There are large numbers of coccidoidal bacilli with varying size (Dia.10-100μm) under epithelia, some of them are phagocytosed by macrophages; some of them are scattering in inflammatory granular tissue. (10×10)

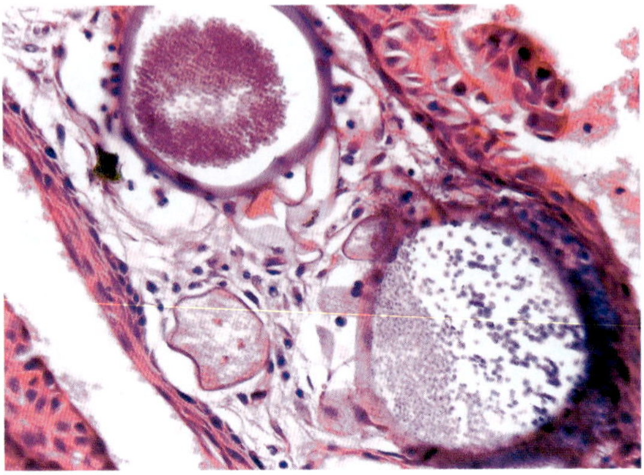

Fig.184 Coccidioidomyocosis (coccidoidal granuloma) of nose (same case as in Fig.183, under high power)

Figure shows: two round and big spores (Dia. about 100μm) with thick capsule. Two of them contain dozens of inner-spores (Dia. about 5μm). If the big spores are broken, the inner-spores would be released in tissue. (10×40)

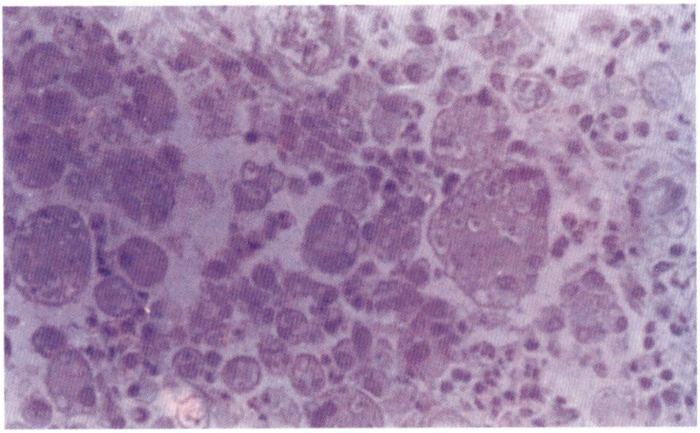

Fig.185 North American blastomycosis of choana (posterior narise)

Male, 26 years old. The neoplasm, which surface was erosional, obstructed his posterior narises.

Figure shows: several polynuclear giant cells, which contain several spores, can be seen in chronic inflammatory granular tissue. Spores, without stained, have round holes in giant cytoplasm. Spores, with stained, have roud and thick capsules under high power lens and make double outlines (Dia. about 8-10μm). Also spores may be scattered in tissue spaces. (10×40)

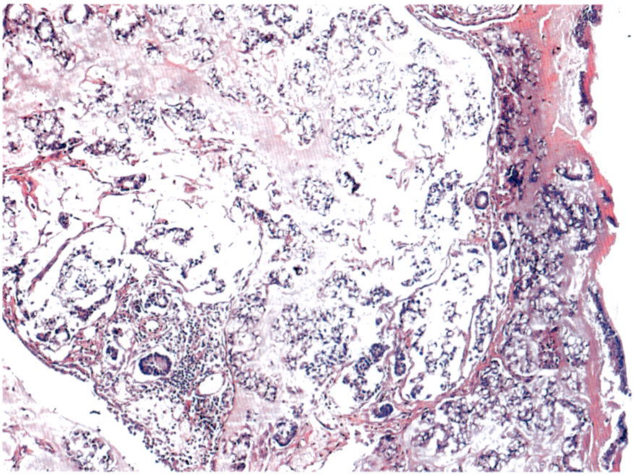

Fig.186 Well-differentiated mucinous adenocarcinoma of nasal cavity

Male, 54 years old. He had the neoplasm in posterior narises, which is greyish with gelatinous section, and the mucus could be scratched out.

Figure shows: some tumor cells arrange in glandular structrue, and part of them are typical columnar adenocarcinoma cells, which secrete large quantity of mucus, mucous lake is formed . (10×10)

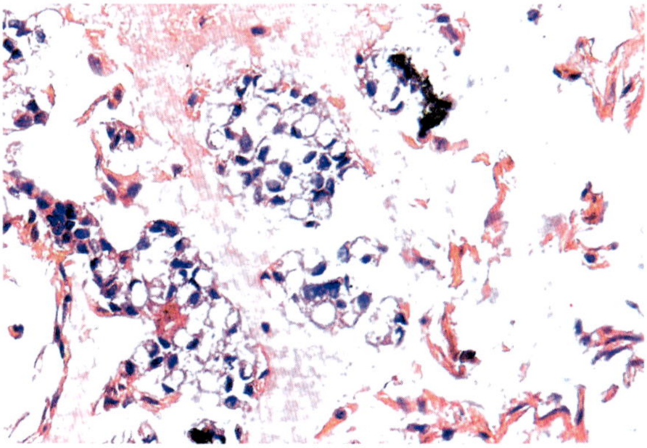

Fig.187 Well-differentiated mucinous adenocarcinoma of nasal cavity (same case as in Fig.186,under high power)

Figure shows: most of tumor cells are swollen.The nuclei are pushed to one side,which so-called signet-ring cells.Mucus of some tumor cells is crushed into peripheral tissue, and in which mucous lake is formed. (10×40)

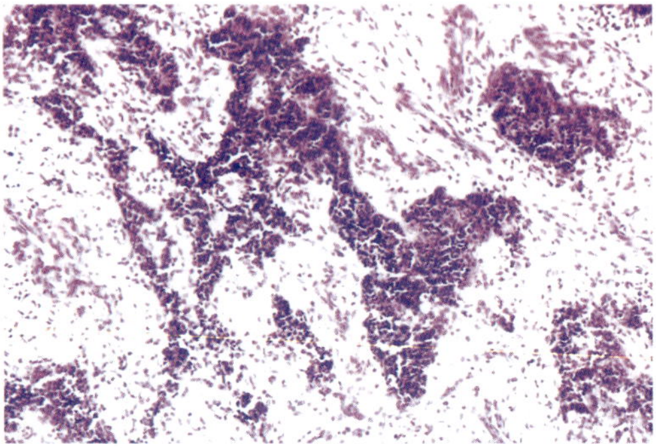

Fig.188 Olfactory neuroblastoma of nose and nasopharynx (also called olfactory esthesioneuroepithelioma)

Male, adult. He had intermittent nasal hemorrhage for four months more,with enlarged left jugular lymph node ($1.0 \times 0.8 \times 0.5cm^3$), without tenderness. Clinic examination: The neoplasm of left posterior naris can be seen, which is corverd by secretory marerials and bleeding easily as palpation. Surgery indicated: The neoplasm with easy hemorrhage and unclear border, grew from ethmoidal foramen with erosional root.

Figure shows: small and round tumor cells have a lobular pattern, separated by vascular fibrous stroma. (10×10)

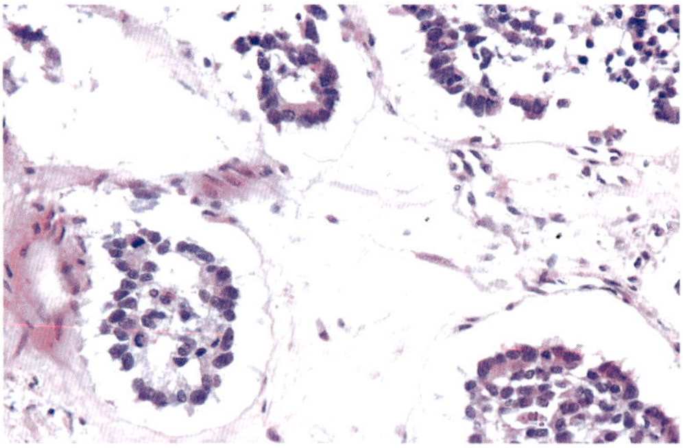

Fig.189 Olfactory neuroblastoma of nose and nasopharynx (same case as in Fig.188, under high power)

Figure shows: round or oval nuclei of tumor cells are hyperchromatic, and possess chromatin granules variant sizes. Some tumor cells are arranged in Homer-Wright rosettes, and that is the special character of the tumor. (10×40)

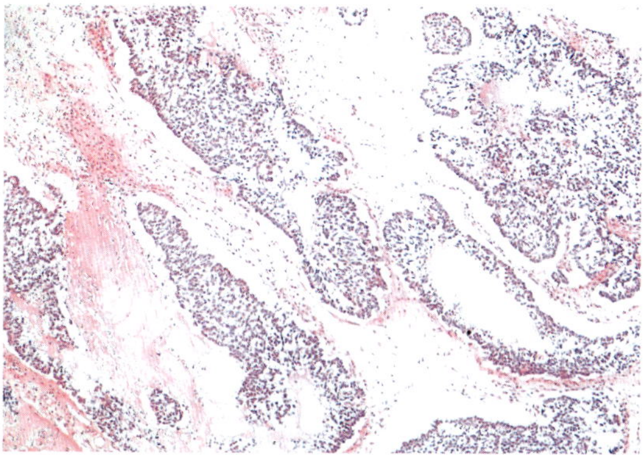

Fig.190 Olfactory neuroblastoma of nose and nasopharynx (also called olfactory esthesioneuroepithelioma)

Female, 13 years old. She had right facial tumescence for four months, and became enlargement quickly near two weeks. The lump (6×5×5cm^3)could be touched in her right face. The neoplasm filled up right nasal cavity, and extended to the palate and gum.

Figure shows: small and round tumor cells have a lobular pattern separated by a connective tissue. (10×10)

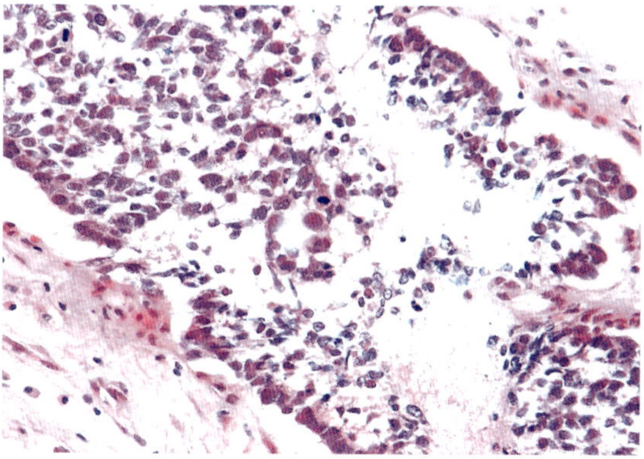

Fig.191 Olfactory neuroblastoma of nose and nasopharynx (same case as in Fig.190, under high power)

Figure shows: a typical Homer-Wright rosettes and the communication of neuroprotofibrillary structure and the tumor cells can be seen. (10×40)

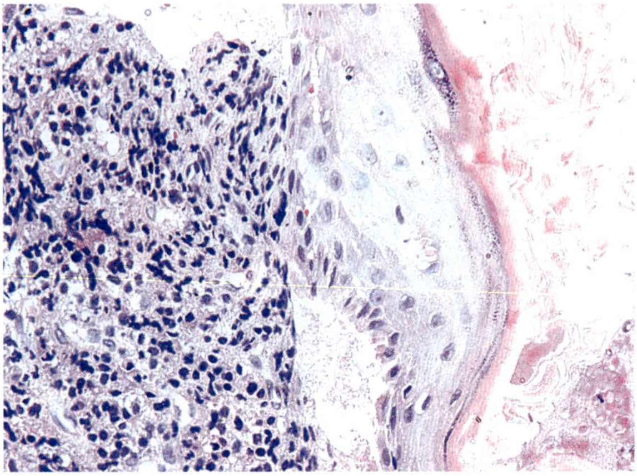

Fig.192 Olfactory neuroblastoma of nose and nasopharynx

Male 29 years old. He had left nasal obstruction and intermittent hemorrhage for three months.

Figure shows: the epithelia of olfactory area have atypical hyperplasia, and transit to transition zone of olfactory neuroblastoma. This indicated the case is originatd from the olfactory mucosa epithelia. (10×40)

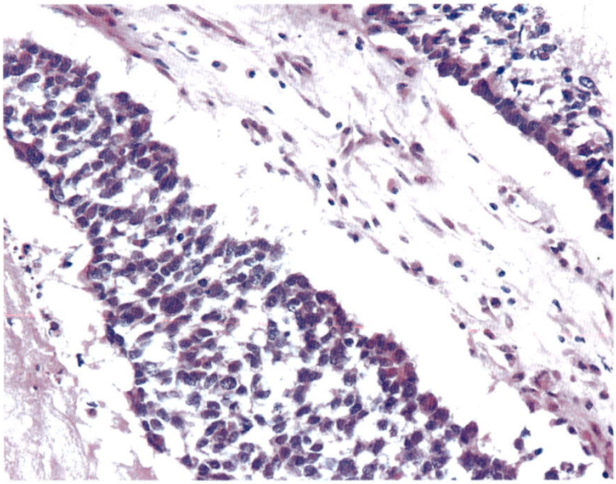

Fig.193 Olfactory neuroblastoma of nose and nasopharynx (another type)

Male, 32 years old. Figure shows: the tumor cells are arranging in cords or columns, and Homer-Wright rosettes still can be seen . (10×40)

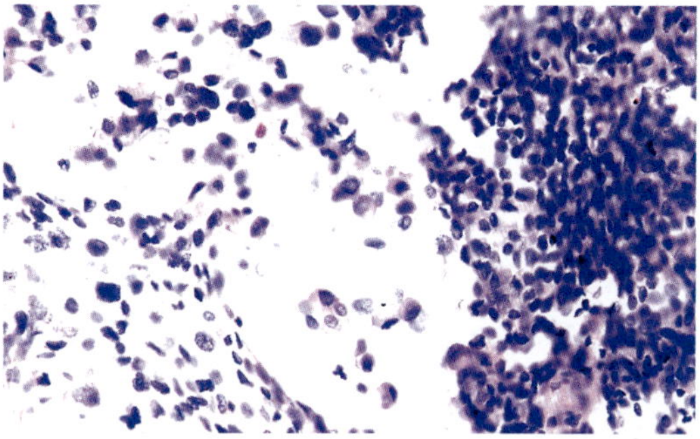

Fig.194 Olfactory neuroblastoma of nose and nasopharynx

Male, adult. The patient had intermittent nasal hemorrhage for eight months, and with the neoplasm of right nasal cavity projecting out of vestibule. He had a surgery in some hospital of Guandong. The biopsy was: malignant tumor. And then radiotherapy had been done, but had no effect. Later, he had a surgery again. Gross specimen is soft, pinkish-grey, like mulberries.

Figure shows: small and round tumor cells with hyperchromatic nuclei and scanty cytoplasm. Part of them connects with fibrils. A cluster of gangliocytes can be seen in the Figue,and this may be indicated the case probably originates from sphenopalatine ganglia. (10×20)

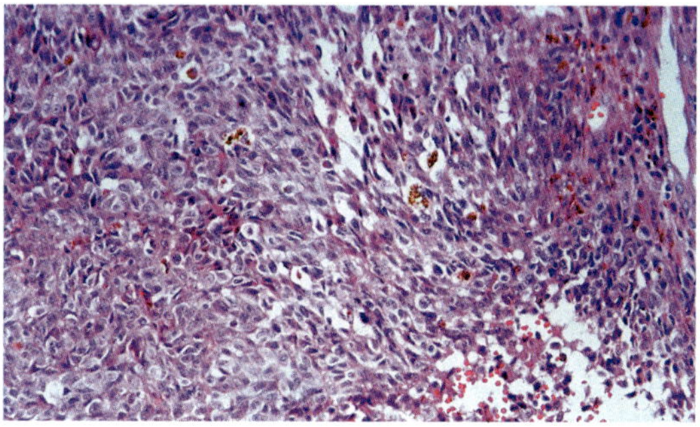

Fig.195 Malignant melanoma of nose

Male, 46 years old. He had gradually nasal obstruction for one year, with intermittent hemorrhage. Examination: the neoplasm of right nasal cavity was putrefactive, putrid and its texture was tough.

Figure shows: diffuse tumor cells infiltrate under nasal mucusal epithelia. The tumor cells are spindle or polygonal. (10×20)

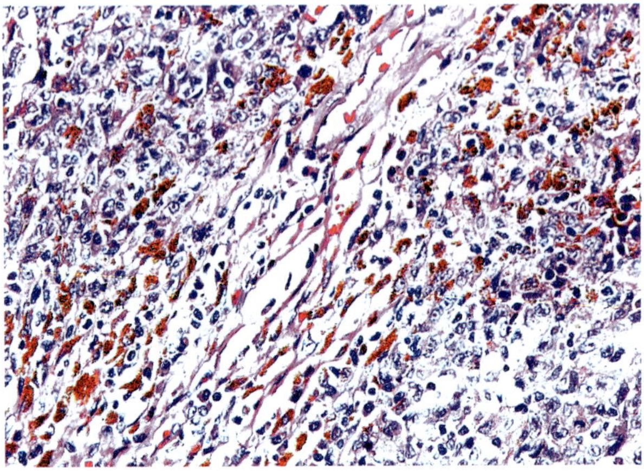

Fig.196 Malignant melanoma of nose
(same case as in Fig.195, under high power)

Figure shows: the tumor cells are polygonal, oval or spindle, and diffusely distribute in lamina propria of nasal mucosa, some of them containing melanin granules. Parts of tumor cells are small and spindle, also containing melanin granules. (10×20)

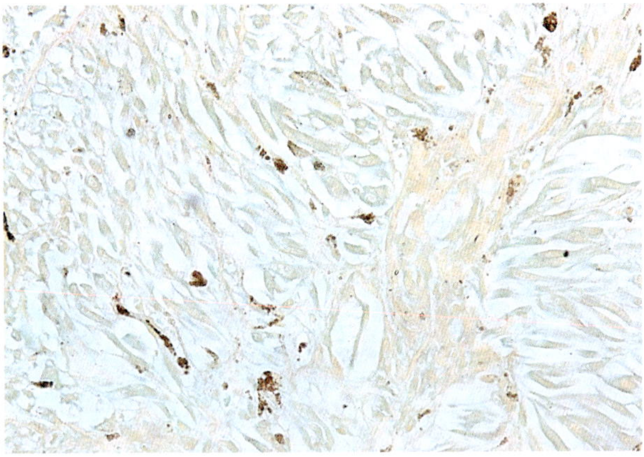

Fig.197 Malignant melanoma of nose
(same case as in Fig.196, another field)

Figure shows: positive melanin staining is prominent in the figue. (ferrous sulfate stain of Lillie's method) (10×40)

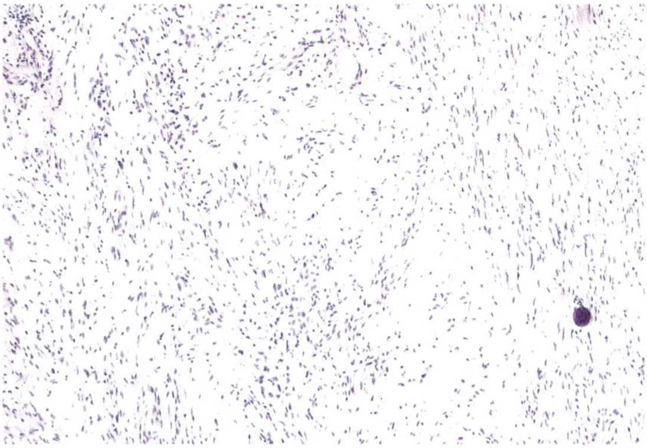

Fig.198 Meningioma of nose and nasopharynx

Female, 25 years old. She had tinnitus of the right ear for half a year, and had the right nasal obstruction, hypoacusis of the right ear and hypopsia of the right eye.

The neoplasm of right posterior nasal cavity and right nasopharynx can be seen, and extend to posterior narises.

Figure shows: spindle or oval tumor cells with whirllike and wavy arrangement. The tumor cells have abundant cytoplasm, with small round or oval nuclei. An indigo psammoma body with concentric circles arrangement can be seen in the Fig. (10×10)

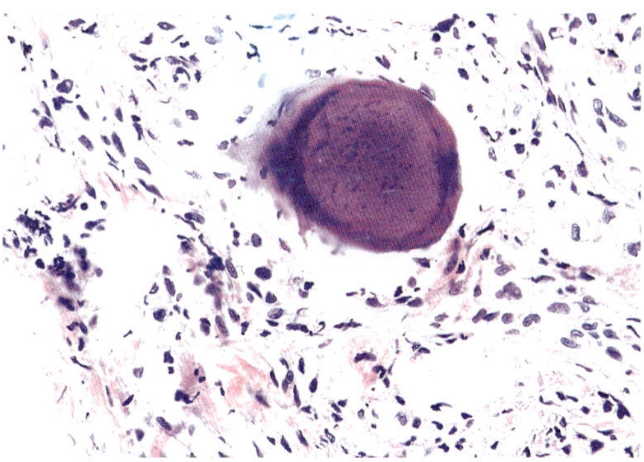

Fig.199 Meningioma of nose and nasopharynx (same case as in Fig.198,another field)

Figure shows: a clear structure of indigo psammoma body can be seen. (10×40)

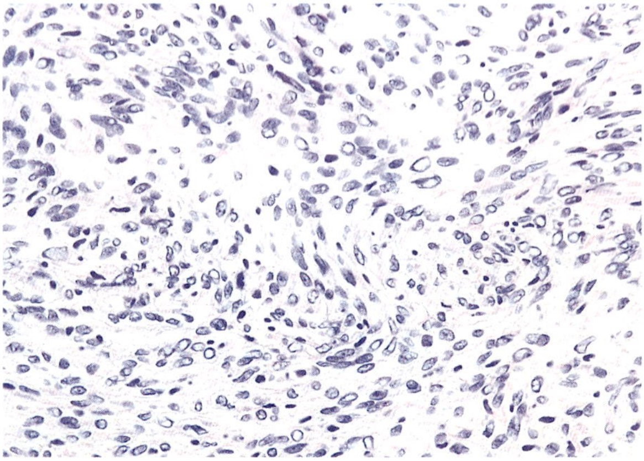

Fig.200 Meningioma of nose and nasopharynx
(same case as in Fig.199,another field)

Figure shows: the tumor cells are obvious spindle, with whirllike arrangement.

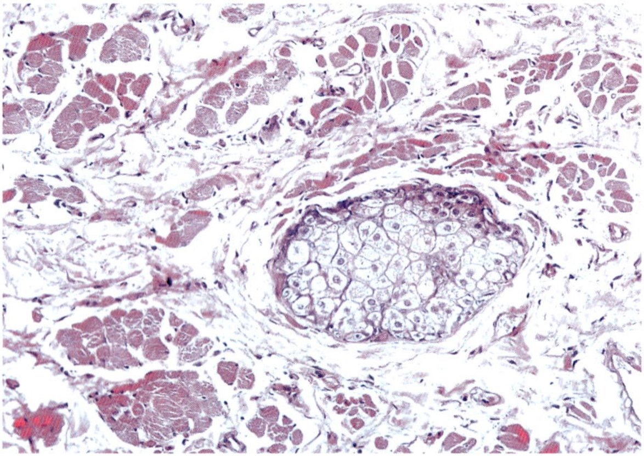

Fig.201 Hamartoma of right nasal vestibule

Male,21 years old.The neoplasm with clear border $(0.8\times0.5\times0.6cm^3)$of right nasal vestibule can be seen.

Figure shows:cross sections of striated muscles,sebaceous glands and surrounded fibrous tissue, above tissue are maturely differentiate, but appear abnormal arrangement and structure. Hamartoma belongs to histiomoid teratogenesis, but is not real tumor. (10×40)

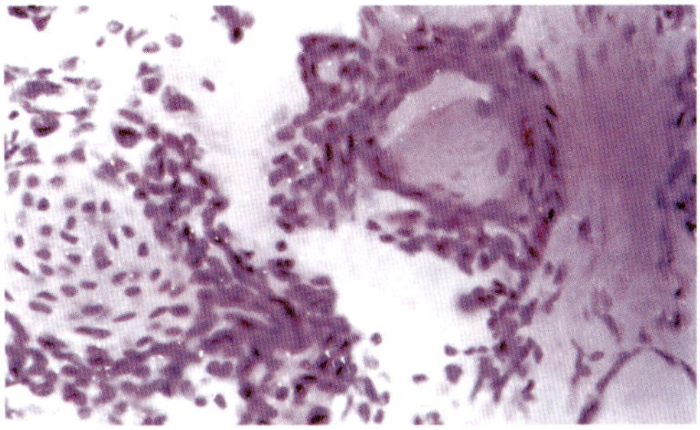

Fig.202 Mixed tumor of nose (salivary gland type)

Female, 53 years old. She had nasal obstruction for 40 years, with nasal back enlargement, the right larger than the left. Her narises were both obstructed. Her palate bones were collapsed. The neoplasm was grayish white and nodular, with smooth surface.

Figure shows: part of the tumor cells are chondroid tissue composed of myoepithelia cells. Parts of them are glandular epithelia, and arrange in masses, with round and hyperchromatic nuclei, scanty cytoplasm and unclear border. There is fibrous tissue with hyaline degeneration in the masses. (10×40)

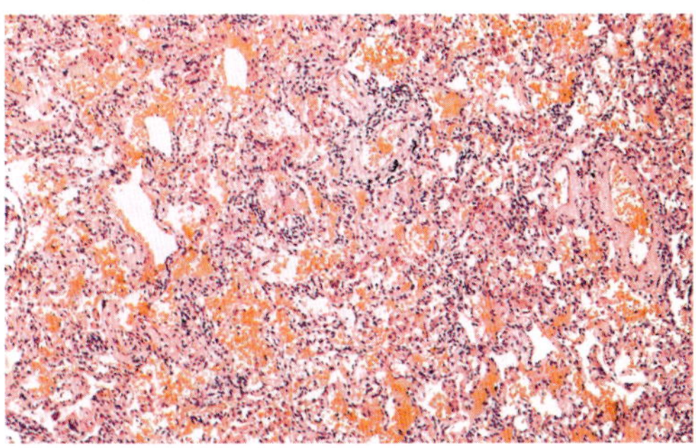

Fig.203 Capillary hemangioma of left nasal cavity

Male, 15 years old. He had hemorrhage of left naris and nasal obstruction for two months.

Examination: the neoplasm (0.6×0.5×1cm^3)of left naris has a pedicle, with smooth surface,flush, easy hemorrhage by palpation.The neoplasm came from nasal septum.

Figure shows: the tumor is composed of uncountable capillaries, and vascular endothelium hyperplasia. (10×10)

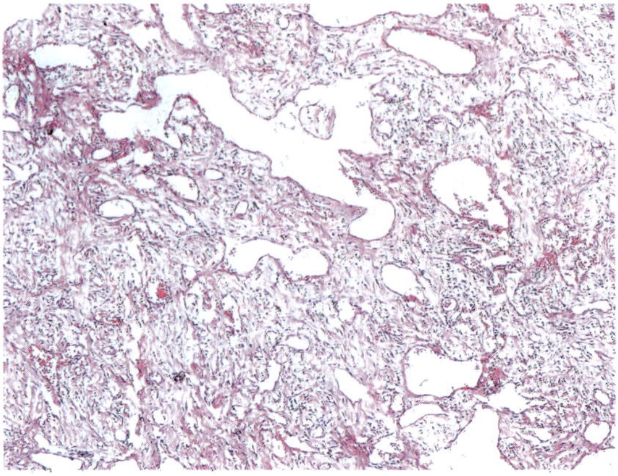

Fig.204 Cavernous hemangioma of nose

Male, 15 years old. Figure shows: the tumor is composed of blood sinuses which are filled up by red blood cells. (10×10)

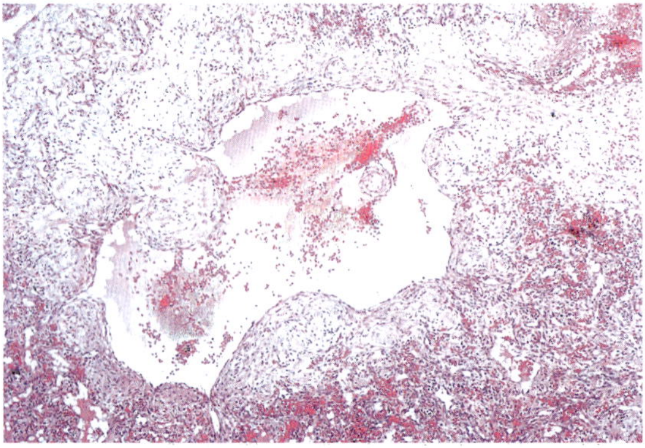

Fig.205 Mixed type hemangioma of nose

Female, 21 years old. She had repeated nasal hemorrhage for one year more, and had nasal obstruction one month ago.Examination:the nasal neoplasm(3.5×3.2×3.0cm^3)was carmine, and easy hemorrhage by palpation.

Figure shows: except capillaries, the tumor is composed of thick-wall veins, with smooth muscle hyperplasia of vessel wall, thickening and irrupting into cavities. (10×10)

6.Addendum 1

Fig.206–208: the sketches of anatomic methods of nasopharynx

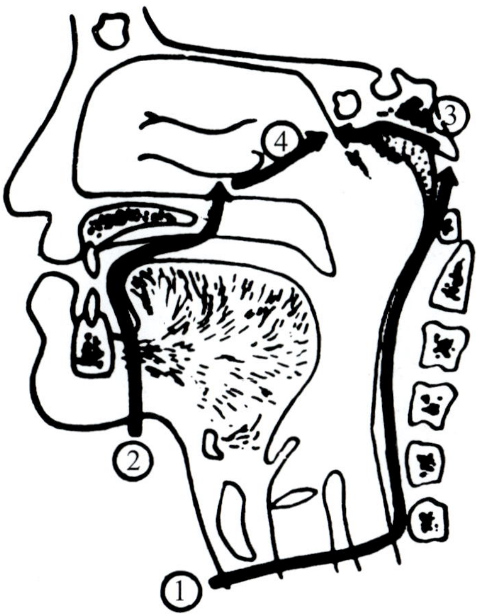

Fig.206 Sketch of sagittal section of skull

Arrow indicates: the order of taking out the whole nasopharynx.

(1)Firstly, cut off trachea and esophagus below larynx, and then peel off esophagus and posterior walls of the whole pharynx, as fingered by arrow ①;

(2)Cut off floor of mouth, epiglottic cartilage(soft oral lid), as fingered by arrow ②. Also cut off the soft tissue of bilateral tongue and pharynx;

(3)Separate (curved scissors) posterior and parietal walls of nasopharynx from base of skull, as fingered by arrow ③;

(4)Snip nasal mucosa at posterior narises, as fingered by arrow④.

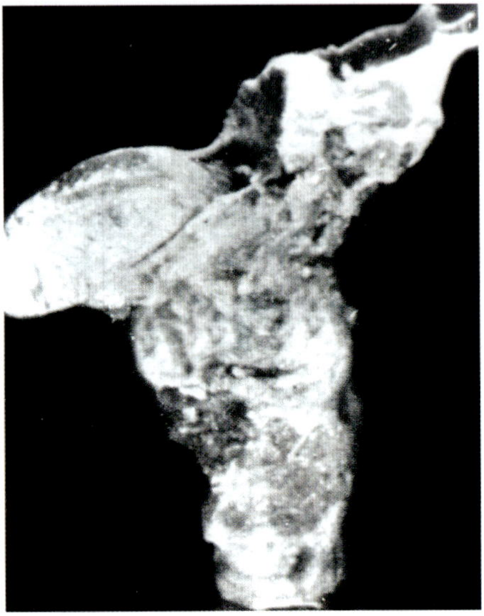

Fig.207 Specimen involved the whole part of nasopharynx, lingua and larynx

Figure shows: taking out specimens of the whole nasopharynx, tongue and pharynx, according to Fig.206 anatomic method.

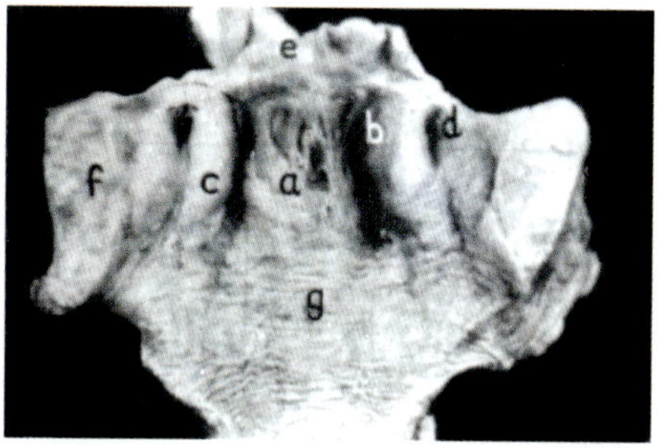

Fig.208 Specimen showing the inner side of a normal nasopharynx

Figure shows: cut off the midline of oral and laryngeal pharynx along root of tongue, and snip the midline of soft palate. Inside of the whole normal nasopharynx (including oral pharynx) can be observed. We can study the early lesions of NPC and transition morphosis of canceration by using the section of all parts of tissue.

Figure shows: (a) pharyngeal tonsils; (b) Rosen–Műller's fossa; (c) Protuberance; (d) pharyngeal opening of eustachian tube; (e) posterior narises; (f) epiglottic cartilage (soft oral lid); (g) oral pharynx.

(Above Fig.207 208 anatomy NO.5345, female, 32 years old, not died from NPC)

7.Addendum 2

Fig.209–211The sketches of the distribution of pseudostratified ciliated columnar epithelia with its transition zone, and squamous cell island, in normal nasopharyngeal mucosa.

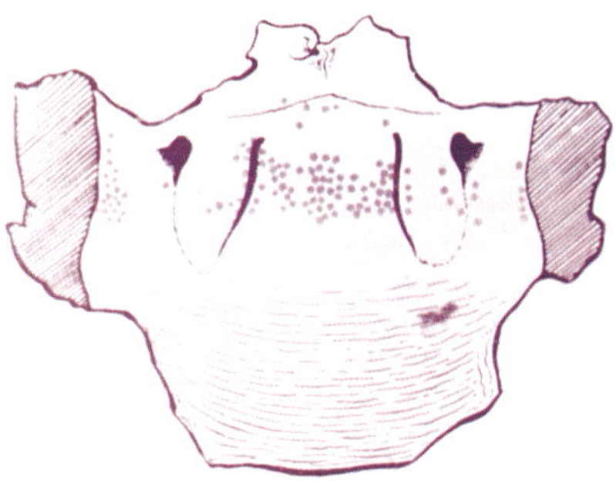

Fig.209 Sketch of showing distribution of squamous cell islands in upper and middle portions of normal nasopharyngeal mucosa in 31 cases

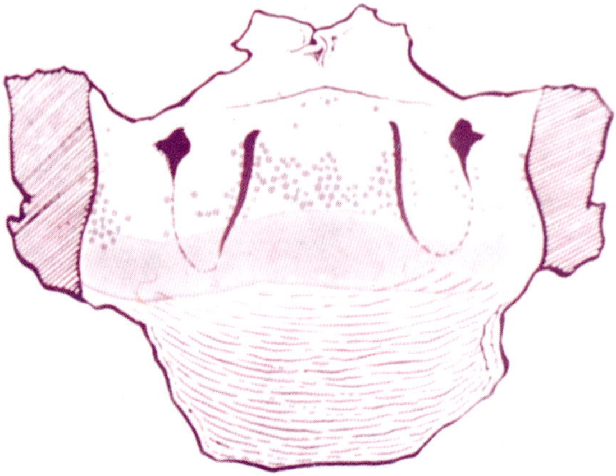

Fig.210 Sketch of showing distribution of squamous cell islands at the epithelium transitional area and the upper portion of nasopharyngeal mucosa

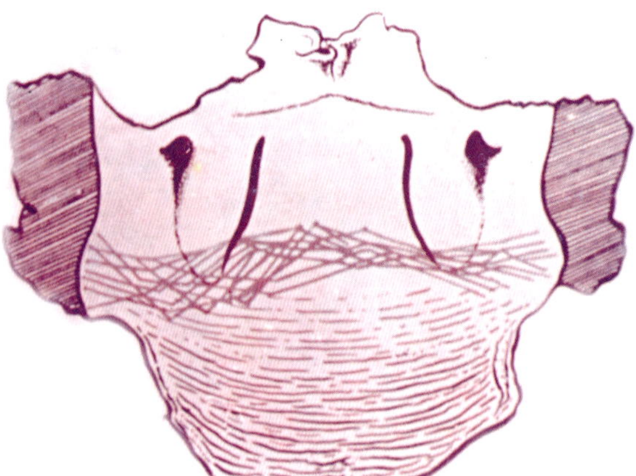

Fig.211 Sketch of showing the distribution of epithelial transitional areas at nasopharyngeal mucosa in 12 cases